Clinical Anesthesia

D0791021

Clinical Anesthesia
Near Misses and Lessons Learned

John G. Brock-Utne, MD, PhD, FFA(SA)

Professor of Anesthesia, Stanford University Medical Center, Stanford, California, USA

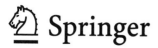 Springer

John G. Brock-Utne, MD, PhD, FFA(SA)
Professor of Anesthesia
Stanford University Medical Center
Stanford, CA 94305-5640
USA

Library of Congress Control Number: 2007930542

ISBN: 978-0-387-72519-2   e-ISBN: 978-0-387-72525-3

Printed on acid-free paper.

© 2008 Springer Science+Business Media, LLC.
All rights reserved. This work may not be translated or copied in whole or in part without the
written permission of the publisher (Springer Science+Business Media, LLC, 233 Spring Street,
New York, NY 10013, USA), except for brief excerpts in connection with reviews or scholarly
analysis. Use in connection with any form of information storage and retrieval, electronic
adaptation, computer software, or by similar or dissimilar methodology now known or here-
after developed is forbidden.
The use in this publication of trade names, trademarks, service marks, and similar terms, even
if they are not identified as such, is not to be taken as an expression of opinion as to whether
or not they are subject to proprietary rights.
While the advice and information in this book are believed to be true and accurate at the date
of going to press, neither the authors nor the editors nor the publisher can accept any legal
responsibility for any errors or omissions that may be made. The publisher makes no warranty,
express or implied, with respect to the material contained herein.

9 8 7 6 5 4 3 2 1

springer.com

For the next generation:
Matthew B., Tobias J., Anders C. Brock-Utne.

Foreword

How do physicians learn to respond to unfamiliar, unusual situations? Medical textbooks are full of helpful information, but they usually do not address complex clinical scenarios. For anesthesiologists, problems are often encountered in the operating room where textbooks and medical journals are not readily available. Even when a text is handy, practical decisions often must be made immediately. Residents in training, recent graduates, and even the most senior anesthesiologists, learn by experience. Case conferences and grand rounds are held in almost every hospital so that all staff members can share in their colleague's experiences. In this book, a companion to *Near Misses in Pediatric Anesthesia*, which was originally published in 1999, John G. Brock-Utne presents a variety of interesting cases. Dr. Brock-Utne has a unique talent for describing real clinical dilemmas and their solutions in a concise, interesting, and entertaining manner. I have known the author for more than 30 years, and his enthusiasm for teaching our residents and medical students, combined with his outstanding abilities as a clinical anesthesiologist, are legendary at Stanford Medical Center. Those same qualities are evident in this book. I believe every reader, from the novice anesthesiologist to the most senior clinician, will benefit from the "experiences" Dr. Brock-Utne brings to this book.

Jay B. Brodsky, MD
Professor (Anesthesia)
Medical Director – Perioperative Services
Stanford University Medical Center
Stanford, CA

Preface

As anesthesiologists we face from time to time difficult decisions in "near miss" situations. The risk/benefit ratios in these cases are often unknown. The near misses reported in this book come mainly from my over 35 years of experience in clinical anesthesia in Scandinavia, South Africa, and the United States.

Each of the 62 cases first gives the reader all of the information necessary to prevent a potential disaster. The following sections provide solutions and discussions of the problem, make recommendations, and provide references for further reading.

Some of the sequences in the management of these cases may be controversial. As such, they may form the basis for a teaching discussion between faculty members and residents in training in anesthesiology. But most of all, this book is designed to alert the reader to various precarious situations that can arise in anesthesia practice in both sophisticated or rural anesthetic environment and how to best prevent and/or deal with them.

These are my lessons learned.

John G Brock-Utne, MD, PhD, FFA(SA)

Acknowledgments

I would like to acknowledge my many colleagues around the world who have contributed to this book through our case reports:

Craig T. Albanese, Karim Ali, Anthony D. Andrews, Derek Ardendorff, Don Armstrong, Pat Bolton, Arne Brock-Utne, Jay B. Brodsky, Michael W. Brook, Greg Botz, John L. Chow, Anne Chowet, Larry F. Chu, Anthony Chung, Michael Cochran, Jeremy S. Collins, John Cummings, Charles DeBattista, Tom G.B. Dow, John W. Downing, Michael F. Dillingham, George E. Dimopoulos, Paul Eckinger, Mark Eggen, Michael Ennis, Gary S. Fanton, Marit Farstad, Steve P. Fischer, Louis Furukawa, Monica Gertsner, Cosmin Guta, Gordon Haddow, Kyle Harrison, James M. Healzer, Bruce Henderson, Rex Henderson, Jerome Hester, Jeff P. Holden, Terry Homer, David Humphrey, Paul Husby, Richard A. Jaffe, Michael Keating, Mai-Elin Koller, Vivek Kulkarni, Andrew Kim, Harry J.M. Lemmens, Phoebe Leith, Richard M. Levitan, Sanford Littwin, Jaimie R. Lopes, T. Lund, Alex Macario, Anne Marie Mallat, Steve J. Manos, Ed R. Mariano, James B. Mark, Mike G. Moshal, Clint Naiker, Cameron Nezhat, Ola J. Ohm, Einar Ottestad, David Parris, Andrew J. Patterson, Diane Pond, Emily Ratner, Joe Roberson, Beemeth Robles, Joe Rubin, Larry J. Saidman, Robert Sanborn, Cliff A. Schmiesing, Daniel S. Seidman, Lars Segadal, Steve Ternlund, Patsy Tew, Phillip R. Torralva, Ken S. Truelsen, Winston C. Vaughan, Steve Welman, Mark Vierra, Debbie M. Williams, Russell K. Woo, Andy A. Sumaran, and Gina Zisook.

I am also greatly indebted to the following:

Dr. Jay B. Brodsky for so kindly agreeing to write a foreword for this book. He is a wonderful friend and a superb and talented anesthesiologist. Stanford University's Department of Anesthesiology is indeed fortunate to have such an outstanding colleague.

Bernadett Romo, secretary in the Department of Anesthesia at Stanford University School of Medicine, for unfailing good humor and dedication to her job.

Stacy Hague and Beth Campbell, both of Springer, and Barbara Chernow and Kathy Cleghorn, both of Chernow Editorial Services, for all of their support and encouragement.

Last, but not least, to my wife Sue, our boys, their wives, and our three grandboys.

John G. Brock-Utne, MD, PhD, FFA(SA)

Contents

1
No Fiberoptic Intubation System: A Potential Problem

You are to anesthetize a 19-yr-old Indian woman (42 kg) who is otherwise healthy, but is coming in for the removal of a large keloid scar (7 cm × 8 cm) on the front of her neck. This was caused 2 yr before by hydrochloric acid (HCl). She tried to drink it in an attempt to commit suicide. Someone prevented her from doing so, but during the tussle that ensued, the large cup of HCl spilt down the front of her neck causing a severe third degree burn. She survived, but is now left with a large keloid scar that has pulled her chin down so that it nearly touches the sternum, and she can only open her mouth slightly (0.5 cm between the top and bottom teeth). You see this young woman in the preoperative area and decide that an awake nasal or oral fiberoptic intubation is needed. Unfortunately, there is no scope available, and the surgeon tells you that if we don't do it today the young woman will not come back. You decide to proceed and take her back to the operating room after an IV is started and 1 mg of midazolam. After routine monitors are placed, you attempt an inhalation induction with sevoflurane, to be followed by a blind oral or nasal endotracheal intubation. Unfortunately, you lose her airway during the induction and she stops breathing. The saturation falls to 82%. You turn the sevoflurane off and attempt to ventilate with 100% oxygen, but with great difficulty. With the sevoflurane off, she slowly begins to breathe again and her saturation improves. Your attempt at an awake nasal intubation also fails. There is no other airway equipment available, e.g., a Trachlight (Laerdal Medical A/S, Stavanger, Norway). You suggest to the surgeon that he does a tracheostomy under local. The surgeon says that will be impossible, as there are no landmarks and it is very difficult to anesthetize the keloid scar with local anesthesia. More important is the fact that the tracheotomy will be in the surgical site, and therefore it is not an option. You attempt to place the smallest pediatric laryngeal mask airway (LMA) that you can find. Unfortunately, even that LMA is too big. In desperation, you now try to pass a pediatric gum-elastic bougie blindly into her trachea both through the mouth and nose. This also fails. Understandably, she is now getting very upset and agitated. The surgeon looks at you and wonders if anything else can be done to secure the airway without doing a tracheostomy. What will you suggest?

Solution

Many years ago, in 1973, at King Edward 8 hospital in Durban, South Africa, Dr. Derek Ardendorf, who is a plastic surgeon, and I were confronted with this problem. An inhalational induction failed, and Dr. Ardendorf chose not to do an elective tracheostomy for the reasons mentioned. So what did we do? I gave the patient the following drugs intravenously: diazepam 5 mg, followed by atropine 0.6 mg and ketamine 2 mg/kg. With the patient asleep, but breathing, the surgeon cut away at the keloid, making it possible for me to extend her neck and open her mouth. When I could get the laryngoscope in the mouth and saw the epiglottis, I gave succinylcholine 40 mg and secured the airway. Hemostatis was achieved, and the surgery was completed successfully. I kept an eye on the patient's future development, and she did very well. The last time I heard from her, she had gotten married.

Discussion

To put this problem more in perspective, in those days, cases such as this were done without oximetry, capnography, or an automated noninvasive blood pressure machine. However, we had electrocardiogram machines in most rooms. Furthermore, there were no pediatric gum-elastic bougies or LMAs. The LMA was introduced into the United States in 1990.

Recommendation

In difficult cases like these, it is imperative that you and the surgeon agree on a plan and, preferably, have a plan B and C. Furthermore, you must have confidence in your colleague's ability, as well as your own.

2
Is the Patient Extubated?

An otherwise healthy 48-year-old man is being ventilated in the intensive
care unit (ICU) after major abdominal surgery. You are called urgently
because the ICU nurse informs you that she can hear air escaping from the
patient's mouth. She is concerned that the patient may have become extubated. His vital signs are HR 90 BP 140/90. Oxygen saturation is 96% on
FiO2 of 100%. You arrive and find him somewhat sedated, but agitated. You
talk to him, but he does not answer back, despite trying to do so. The nurse
tells you that the patient was previously saturating at 92–94% on 40% FiO2.
The ventilator is alarming. The endotracheal tube (ETT) (#8) is taped at
22 cm. A universal bite block (B&B Medical Technologies, Vista, CA) is seen
in his mouth (Fig. 2.1). The bite block consists of a 5-cm-long hollow plastic
tube that has a 0.5-cm-long longitudinal opening. This opening stretches
from top to bottom going through the entire length of the bite block. An
anchoring device (a plastic strap) is available on the bite block to attach it
to the ETT. An audible leak is heard. You detach him from the ventilator,
and with an Ambu bag you confirm that he has bilateral air entry, although
they are distant. Air/bubbles can be heard/seen coming from his mouth. You
decide to blow up the ETT cuff, as there must be a leak caused by lack of air
in the ETT cuff. However, the cuff on the pilot tubing is already blown up
and feels very tight. You push some more air into the pilot tubing. No
improvement is seen and you can still hear a leak at the mouth. The ventilator continues to alarm. What will you do and what is the cause of your
dilemma?

Solution

Because you believe there must be something wrong with the cuff and/or
pilot tubing, you exchange the existing ETT with a new ETT using a gum
elastic bougie (1). The cuff on the new ETT is blown up, and no more leaks
are heard. The patient is sedated, and the ventilator now works without

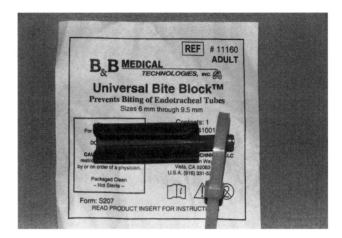

FIGURE 2.1. Universal bite block.

causing alarm. You look at the ETT and the bite block that have been removed in one piece (i.e., they are anchored together with a plastic strap). You see the cause of the problem. The bite block had migrated down the ETT and clamped off the pilot tubing completely (Fig. 2.2). If one had discovered the problem, one could have moved the bite block up the ETT, thereby releasing the obstruction in the pilot tubing (Fig. 2.3).

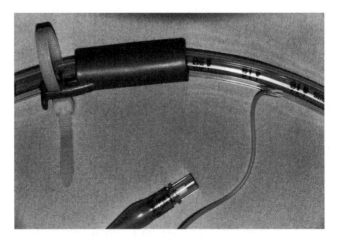

FIGURE 2.2. Bite block seen on ETT.

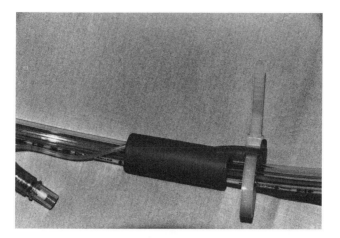

FIGURE 2.3. Bite block shown to clamp-off pilot tubing.

Discussion

This case is similar to a previously described case (2). When faced with an obstructed pilot tubing that causes a leak due to the inability to fill the ETT cuff with air, the correct thing to do is to relieve the obstruction if possible. If that cannot be done, one is forced to replace the ETT. Replacing the ETT may also be considered the safest thing to do, as the original pilot tubing may generate a leak at any time after the obstruction is relieved.

Recommendation

Beware of bite blocks, as they can cause problems.

References

1. Robles B, Hester J, Brock-Utne JG. Remember the gum-elastic bougie at extubation. J Clin Anesth 1993;5:329–331.
2. Brock-Utne AJ. Endotracheal bite block. A word of caution. Anesth Analg 2006;103:495–496.

3
A Strange Computerized Electrocardiogram Interpretation

A 38-yr-old man is scheduled for vasectomy reversal. He is healthy except for a history of several anxiety attacks, after the death of his youngest child, which occurred 6 mo before this procedure. His symptoms included shortness of breath, palpitations, and dizziness. He denies any history of cardiac or neurological disease, syncope, exercise-induced chest symptoms, and any family risk factors for coronary artery disease. He states he is fit, and his wife concurred that he exercises regularly. Because the patient was deemed healthy and not scheduled for major surgery, he was not evaluated in the Anesthesia Preoperative Assessment Clinic before surgery.

On the day of surgery, a full history and examination is done. The history was as already reported, with one general anesthetic for sterilization that had been uneventful. On examination, nothing abnormal was detected. His initial blood pressure was 133/73 mmHg, and the heart rate was 73 sinus rhythm by palpation. Because the patient is concerned that his anxiety symptoms might actually represent a cardiac disorder and no previous electrocardiogram (ECG) had been done, an ECG is ordered. With the patient lying flat, a 20-gauge intravenous catheter is inserted in the back of his right hand. The ECG is done at the same time. The ECG is shown in Figure 3.1. The patient is awake and cooperative, but feels a bit anxious. His blood pressure is 80/50 mmHg, and his heart rate deemed to be regular at 36 beats per min (BPM).

With his history and the result of the computerized ECG, what would you do? Will you proceed or will you cancel the case for further workup by the cardiologist? What will you tell the patient about his ECG?

Solution

A diagnosis of vasovagal reaction was made, and the patient treated with atropine 0.5 mg IV. An ECG repeated 5 min later shows sinus rhythm at a rate of 51 BPM (Fig. 3.2). The patient was evaluated as stable, and he was reassured that this second ECG was normal. He was told that the reason

Rate 35 . ATRIAL FIBRILLATION, VENTRICULAR RATE = 35
PR   . BORDERLINE ST ELEVATION, INFERIOR LEADS
QRSD93 .
QT 438 .
QTc 334

 – –AXIS – –
P
QRS 72   – ABNORMAL ECG –
T   29   PRELIMINARY-MD MUST REVIEW

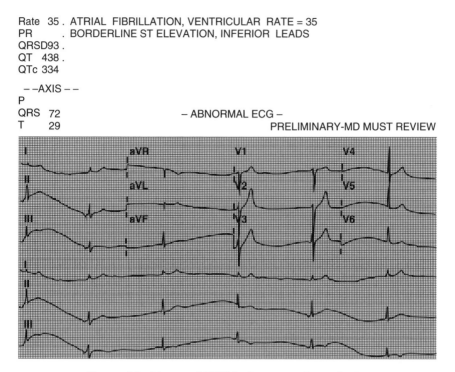

FIGURE 3.1. Abnormal ECG before general anesthesia.

Rate 51 . NORMAL SINUS RHYTHM, RATE 51
PR   150 . ST ELEVATION, PROBABLY NORMAL EARLY REPOLARIZATION VARIANT
QRSD87 .
QT 391 .
QTc 360

 – – AXIS – –
P   35
QRS 19   – OTHERWISE NORMAL ECG –
T   37   PRELIMINARY-MD MUST REVIEW

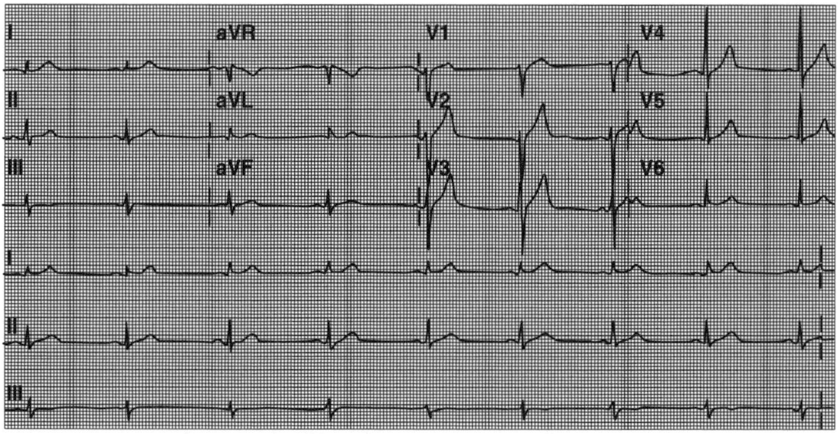

FIGURE 3.2. Normal ECG after vasovagal reaction and treatment with atropine 0.5 mg IV.

for the repeat ECG was that he had had a fainting episode while the IV was being placed. The faint had caused his heart to slow down and give an abnormal ECG tracing. He underwent an uneventful general anesthetic, and two subsequent ECGs done in the postanesthesia care unit (PACU) at 2 and 4 h after the initial abnormal tracing showed sinus rhythm with a normal heart rate and a borderline left axis deviation. His post anesthesia care unit and postdischarge course was uneventful.

Discussion

A similar case has been reported previously (1). Computerized ECG programs have been used in clinical practice for nearly 20 yr. Surprisingly, there is little published data analyzing their accuracy and effect on clinical practice. A study by Jakobsson et al. (2) showed that 82% of computer interpretations were judged to be adequate, versus 64% of the physician's interpretations. Spodnick and Bishop (3) found that computer interpretations of ECGs recorded 1 min apart were significantly and grossly different in 36 out of 92 (39%) unselected pairs of tracings. Of interest here is that atrial fibrillation was the computer interpretation in 11 of the 36 pairs for one tracing, but a totally different rhythm was diagnosed in the second identical tracing. Our case presents several limitations of computer ECG interpretation. Firstly, the machine incorrectly diagnosed atrial fibrillation, although in fact Fig. 3.1 shows two abnormal rhythms present. Broad inverted P waves are seen in two complexes in the rhythm strip from leads II and III (at the bottom of Fig. 3.1), suggesting an ectopic atrial focus. P waves generated by the sinus node should be upright in all leads except V 1, where they may be biphasic (4). Fig. 3.2 shows the return of normal P wave morphology, in which the P waves are upright in all leads. In the remainder of the complexes seen in the rhythm strips from leads II and III (Fig. 3.1), no P waves are present, which is consistent with junctional rhythm. In essence, the computer program misinterpreted the variable rate (because of the alternating presence of two "escape" rhythms) and the absence of P waves in a majority of the complexes as atrial fibrillation.

Should this patient have had an ECG preoperatively a few days before surgery? Roizen recommends not obtaining ECGs in asymptomatic men under the age of 40 yr (5). This is based on the very low incidence of significant abnormalities detected on the preoperative ECG in men under the age of 40 who are asymptomatic and who have had a thorough preoperative evaluation (6). At Stanford, healthy asymptomatic men under the age of 50 do not undergo routine preoperative ECG testing in the Anesthesia Preoperative Assessment Clinic (7). In retrospect, if a preoperative normal ECG had been found, one would not have ordered a repeat preoperative ECG on the day of surgery. As it was, the abnormal ECG, obtained on the day of surgery, did little to reassure him that he was not suffering from some potentially significant cardiac disease. In this case, the computer interpretation was significantly in error and, if not reviewed, could have led to an unnecessary surgical cancellation with possible hospitalization and added stress to the patient. It is important to realize that ECG programs do not consider other pertinent clinical data, like with this relatively fit, anxious, young man with no history of heart disease and who is having an IV started while the ECG tracing was obtained. Atrial fibrillation, with a very slow ventricular response rate, might be expected in a patient with chronic atrial fibrillation and a very high serum digoxin level, or with serious underlying conduction disease.

Recommendation

Computerized ECG results must always be reviewed by the physician and interpreted in light of clinical data.

References

1. Schmiesing CA, Brock-Utne JG, Fischer SP. Misinterpretation by computerized ECG machine – a case report and literature review. Am J Anesthesiol 2001;28: 351–354.
2. Jakobsson A, Ohlin P, Pahlm O. Does a computer-based ECG recorder interpret electrocardiograms more efficiently than physicians? Clin Physiol 1985; 5:417–423.
3. Spodnick DH, Bishop RL. Computer treason, intraobserver variability of an electrocardiographic computer system. Am J Cardiol 1997;80:102–103.
4. Marriot HJL. Practical Electrocardiography. 7th ed. Baltimore, MD: Williams and Wilkins; 1983:102–103.
5. Roizen MF. Preoperative evaluation. In: Miller RD, ed. Anesthesia. 4th ed. New York: Churchill Livingstone; 1994;845–847.
6. Mooreman JR, Hlatky MA, Eddy DM, et al. The yield of the routine admission electrocardiogram. A study in a general medical service. Ann Intern Med 1985;103:590–595.
7. Fischer SP. Development and effectiveness of an anesthesia preoperative evaluation clinic in a teaching hospital. Anesthesiology 1996;85:196–206.

4
Fractured Neck of Femur in an Elderly Patient

An 83-yr-old woman (70 kg and 5'5" tall) is admitted to the emergency room after a fall in her nursing home. She has fractured the neck of her femur, but otherwise there is no trauma. In addition, she has many medical problems, including coronary artery disease, hypertension, and chronic obstructive lung disease. On examination, she was cooperative and orientated for time and place. She has mild to moderate bilateral ankle and sacral edema. HR 100 atrial fibrillation, blood pressure (BP) 170/100. The electrocardiogram (ECG) shows old MI change with left-axis deviation. Room oxygen saturation is 91%. Her chest is clear, except for crepitations at the bases and increased respiratory wheeze. Because she is orientated for time and place, she requests a spinal anesthetic, as she is worried about going to sleep. You are happy to oblige and explain that she must either sit up or lie on her side for you to do the spinal. She absolutely refuses and claims this will be very painful. She has received morphine 10 mg in the emergency room. You attempt to sit her up, but she complains of severe pain. You give her midazolam 0.5 mg and fentanyl 50 mg, slowly. A little later she claims to feel better. However, her oxygen saturation has now fallen to 87% on room air. You give her supplemental oxygen and her saturation improves to 93%. You attempt to sit her up again, but she complains bitterly. You could use a small dose of ketamine so that you can place the spine in a lateral position, but you are concerned about a potentially unacceptable increase in BP with ketamine and the need to use atropine with its side effects. What else could you do to make her pain free, so that you can perform the spinal block?

Solution

You can perform a femoral nerve block.

Discussion

This is a relative easy block to perform, if you do it frequently. I normally do this block as soon as the patient has agreed to a spinal anesthetic for a fractured neck of femur, preferably in the preoperative holding area. By the time the patient arrives in the operating room, the block is working. As for the anatomy: the vein, artery, and nerve lie from medial to lateral. The femoral nerve lies behind and lateral to the vascular sheath and, unlike the vessels, is not within it. All three are deep to the fascia lata, but, unfortunately, the exact position of the femoral nerve in relation to the artery is inconstant. It may be close to the sheath or several centimeters lateral to it. Remember that it is usually more deeply placed. These factors often make the blocking of the nerve more difficult than anticipated. When the sciatic and femoral nerve blocks are combined, the femoral nerve block is the one that most often fails (1). However, the advent of the nerve stimulator does make this block easier. When successful, it provides analgesia for the upper part of the femoral shaft, including the neck. The technique consists of drawing a line between the anterior superior iliac spine and the pubic tubercle (2). This line marks the inguinal ligament. The needle should be inserted just below the ligament and 1 cm lateral to the artery. You may feel a "click" as the needle passes through the fascia lata. If this occurs you should be ascertaining paraesthesia or a nerve twitch with the stimulator. If you are 3–4 cm deep in an average-sized person, you are too deep. Start again, either laterally or medially. I deposit 15–20 ml of lidocaine 1–1.5% and find this to be very satisfactory in most cases. If you don't find the nerve, then inject it in a fanwise fashion, from the artery to a point 3 cm lateral to it.

Recommendation

In these cases, a successful femoral nerve block can be invaluable, and your patients will thank you.

References

1. Moore DC. Regional Block. A Handbook for Use in the Clinical Practice of Medicine and Surgery. 4th ed. Springfield, IL.: Charles C. Thomas; 1965.
2. Wildsmith JAW, Armitage EN. Principles and Practice of Regional Anesthesia. 2nd ed. Churchill Livingstone; 1993.

5
Spinal Anesthetic That Wears Off Before Surgery Ends

A 68-yr-old woman, previously healthy, is scheduled for a large inguinal hernia repair. She has a class 3 Mallampati score, weighs 104 kg, and is 5'5" and has GERD (gastro-esophageal reflux disease). She tells you that a previous general anesthetic, not long ago, was complicated by great difficulty in securing the airway with an endotracheal tube. She was advised to tell any future anesthesiologist about this potential problem. She is nervous about a general anesthetic and requests a spinal anesthetic. You place an uneventful spinal at L3-4 with 1.4 ml bupivacaine 0.5%. The spinal works well, and the surgery begins. Operative problems, mainly with lack of proper equipment, are encountered and the procedure that should have taken 30 min is now at 2 h and still ongoing. The patient begins to complain of pain. You give some sedation with midazolam up to 2 mg and fentanyl up to 75 mg, while the surgeon injects into the surgical site and around with 50 ml of lidocaine 1%. Neither has much effect, as the patient still complains of pain and looks irritated by the whole proceedings. You consider an awake fiberoptic intubation, followed by a general anesthetic. Unfortunately, you are now told that all fiberoptic intubation equipment are being serviced and won't be back before tomorrow. You dismiss the idea of more sedation and of inducing general anesthesia via facemask as too dangerous. The surgeon who is a friend of yours, and usually very reliable with his estimated surgical time, tells you that he will be only 10–15 min. You believe him, but what are you to do?

Solution

You ask the patient to take 30 ml of oral Bicitra (an antacid), which she does. Metoclopramide 10 mg IV is also given before giving atropine 05 mg (1) and ketamine 1–2 mg/kg IV. In these cases, ketamine can be a real winner, as respiration is not depressed, except in large doses (1). An adequate surgical anesthesia is established, and the surgeon completes his case. He is very grateful.

Discussion

The prevention of aspiration cannot be guaranteed with the use of ketamine without safeguarding the airway. Where there is a risk of aspiration, an oral antacid and IV metoclopramide should be considered. Both drugs also increase the lower esophageal tone (1,2), and the oral antacid acts by increasing the pH of the stomach (3). A related compound to ketamine is phencyclidine, which was used in anesthesia but withdrawn because of the high incidence of hallucination (4). It is, however, still used in animals. An intravenous dose of 2 mg/kg of ketamine will produce anesthesia in 30 s and last for 5–10 min. An i.m. dose of 10 mg/kg results in anesthesia in 3–4 min, lasting 10–20 min. Remember that you must always use a drug like benzodiazepines and/or droperidol before ketamine, to reduce the incidence of emergence sequelae (4). These include postoperative disorientation, confusion, and irrational behavior. Auditory and visual hallucinations are common. Visual hallucinations with terrifying dreams are, in the author's opinion, much more common than auditory problems (5,6). When ketamine was first introduced in 1965 by Domino et al. (7), this was a real problem until a remedy suggested by Dundee et al. (8), using an opiate-hyoscine premedication, decreased the incidence. However, small amounts of benzodiazepines are more effective. Excess salvation with the use of ketamine can also be a problem and glycopyrrolate or atropine may be required.

Recommendation

Remember ketamine in these cases, as it can be a real "lifesaver."

References

1. Brock-Utne JG, Rubin J, Downing JW, Dimopoulos GE, Moshal MG, Naicker M. The administration of metoclopramide with atropine. A drug interaction effect on the gastro-oesoephageal sphincter in man. Anaesthesia 1976;31:1186–1190.
2. Brock-Utne JG, Dow TGB, Welman S, Dimopoulos GE, Moshal MG. The effect of metoclopramide on the lower oesophageal sphincter in late pregnancy. Anaesth Intensive Care 1978;6:26–29.
3. Brock-Utne JG, Downing JW. The lower oesaphageal sphincter and the anaesthetist. S Afr Med J 1986;70:170–171.
4. Kohrs R, Durieux ME. Teaching an old drug new tricks. Anesth Analg 1998;87: 186–193.
5. Johnstone M, Evans V, Baigel S. Sernyl (CI-395) in clinical anaesthesia. Br J Anaesth 1959;31:433–439.
6. Copple D, Bovill JG, Dundee JW. The taming of ketamine. Anaesthesia 1973;28: 293–296.
7. Domino EF, Chodoff P, Corssen G. Pharmacologic effects of CI-581 a new dissociative anesthetic in man. J Clin Pharmacol 1965;6:279–291.
8. Dundee JW, Bovill JG, Clarke RSJ, Pandit SK. Problems with ketamine in adults. Anaesthesia 1971;26:86.

6
Just a Simple Monitored Anesthesia Care Case

It is the end of a long day in the operating room (OR). You are scheduled to do an emergency Broviac catheter placement under monitored anesthesia care (MAC). The scheduler promises you that this is your last case of the day. The patient is an 83-yr-old female who has been in the hospital for 3 d for a work-up of her severe aortic stenosis for a possible aortic valve replacement. During the work-up she has developed acute renal failure; hence, the Broviac catheter placement. The patient is admitted to the OR from the intensive care unit (ICU) and her consent is signed by her son. Neither he nor any other relative is available before surgery. You meet the patient outside your operating room and the surgeon is anxious to get going. You say that you would like to speak to the patient and examine her. The patient is partially orientated for time and place. She says she understands that she needs the Broviac catheter for a "problem with her kidneys." She is a small lady, weighing 59 kg and 5′6″ tall. She has edema of her legs and sacrum. Her vital signs are HR 110 regular with a blood pressure (BP) of 130/90. Room air oxygen saturation is 91%. The patient is receiving 10 liters/min oxygen via a facemask. Chest auscultation reveals decreased air entry at both bases, with crepitations and rales all over her chest. She has shallow breathing at a rate of 34. Her neck veins are distended. You diagnose congestive cardiac failure and the surgeon concurs with your assessment but wishes to proceed. You elect not to give her any sedation or narcotics except for more furosemide 40 mg IV. The patient is placed on the operating table and you reassure her and place noninvasive monitors. An oxygen mask is placed with a strap on her head, and 8 liters of oxygen is provided. The surgeon injects 20 ml of lidocaine 1% into the surgical site. The junior intern has several attempts at finding the left subclavian vein. Suddenly, there is a major drop in the end-tidal CO_2 from 38 mmHg to 15 mmHg, and oxygen saturation falls to 83%. You provide mask ventilation with 100% oxygen and the patient's saturation goes up to 94%, the highest it has been since you took over her care. You are about to intubate the patient's trachea when the circulating nurse informs you that the patient is a DNR/DNI (do not resuscitate/do not intubate). You elect not to intubate the patient but to continue to mark ventilation. A quick exam of the chest reveals that she has a pneumothorax. Treat her pneumothorax with an emergency chest drain. With the help of the nurse you assemble the drain in less than 1 min (1,2). For further information on making a quick underwater drain, see the Appendix on page 157. With a functioning chest drain and more furosemide, the patient almost returns to her baseline over a period of 10–20 min. The surgeon aborts the catheter placement and the patient is taken back to the ICU. Unfortunately, she dies within 2 h of arriving in the ICU, without any heroic attempts to save her life as per her DNR/DNI.

Shortly after her demise, you manage to meet the patient's three surviving children, a son who is a physician and two daughters who are malpractice lawyers. You explain what happened and they listen politely. At the end you ask them if they have any questions and the one daughter says: "Thank you for taking the time to explain all this to us. We are also grateful that she seemed not to have suffered too greatly. However, I have only one question for you." What do you think the question was?

Solution

The question was "Did you or did you not at any stage during your care put a tube in our mother's windpipe?" I told her "No." She said, "Thank you, doctor that will be all."

Discussion

Do not resuscitate and DNI are orders established by competent patients or an elected health care agent to provide a mechanism for withholding specific resuscitative therapies in the event of a cardiopulmonary arrest. Most surgeries performed in patients with DNR/DNI orders are palliative and designed to improve patient comfort or simplify care. Hence, many individual practitioners and hospitals have made an exception to this covenant and made it routine to suspend these orders the moment the patient enters the OR (3). The fact that the majority of these patients are willing to temporarily forego their DNR status in exchange for an anticipated benefit of surgery, has been challenged by both bioethicists and patient rights advocates (4–7).

My suggestion to reduce conflict and potential liability is the following:

1. Each department of anesthesiology should have a policy regarding DNR orders in the perioperative period (8).

2. Do not routinely assume that the DNR/DNI orders are abandoned for surgery without discussing it with the patient or the patient's health care agent. For instance, a cancer patient who is a DNR may want the DNR lifted for some sort of palliative surgery, but a patient with severe coronary

artery disease may want to keep the DNR order in place for some last ditch, risky cardiac surgery. In either case, it is imperative to inform everyone of what may happen with or without the DNR. The patient or the surrogate must make a decision on how they want the procedure to be done.

3. You may express concern about where to draw the line between anesthesia care and resuscitation that may conflict with the DNR order. It is not for you to make that decision. It is the duty of the patient or the health care agent to tell you. You must attempt at all costs to reach a consensus on how to handle the surgery. Do not proceed before it is reached.

4. It is important to write in the chart, before the surgery, something like this: "Discussed the risks and benefits of surgery with and without DNR, including the risk that resuscitation may inadvertently occur. Patient understands there is no guarantee about outcome. Patient/ health care agent wishes to proceed with DNR in place or DNR not in place."

The reader is referred to the American Society of Anesthesiologists publication, entitled *Ethical Guidelines for the Anesthesia Care of Patients and Do Not Resuscitate Orders or Other Directives That Limit Treatment* (8).

Recommendation

In our specialty, the patient's autonomy is honored through the process of informed consent, and it is our duty to adhere to what has been mutually agreed upon with or without DNR in place in the OR.

References

1. Brock-Utne JG, Brodsky JB, Haddow G, Mark JB. A simple underwater apparatus for use in emergencies. J Cardiothorac Vasc Anesth 1991;5:195–197.
2. Brock-Utne JG. Near misses in pediatric anesthesia. Butterworth-Heinemann, 1999.
3. Cohen B, Cohen PJ. Do-not-resuscitate order in the operating room. NEJM 1991;325:1879–1882.
4. Keffer KJ, Keffer HI. Do-not-resuscitate in the operating room: moral obligations of anesthesiologist. Anesth Analg 1992;74:901–905.
5. Miller RB. Do not resuscitate orders in the operating room: a topic whose time has come. Semin Anesth 1991;12:295–303.
6. Truog RD. "Do not resuscitate " orders during anesthesia and surgery. Anesthesiology 1991;74:606–608.
7. Younger SJ, Cascorbe HF, Shuck JM. DNR in the operating room, not really a paradox. JAMA 1991;266:2433–2434.
8. Margolis JO, McGrath BJ, Kussin PS, Schwinn DA. Do not resuscitate (DNR) orders during surgery: Ethical Foundation for Institutional Policies in the United States. Anesth Analg. 1995;80:806–809.
9. Fine PG. DNR in the OR- anesthesiologist medical ethics and guidelines. ASA Newsletter 1994;58:10–14.

7
Smell of Burning in the Operating Room

A 65-yr-old man (American Society of Anesthesiologists physical status 2) is undergoing a transurethral resection of the prostate under spinal anesthesia. Adequate regional anesthesia is established, and no sedation is given at the patient's request. Nasal oxygen at 2 liters/min is provided throughout the procedure. The surgeon encounters difficulty in passing the urethral scope. He disconnects the fiberoptic illumination system (FIS) and leaves it over the level of the pubic symphysis. A few minutes later the patient tells you, "I seem to smell burning." You can't smell anything but after putting your nose near the patient's head you also smell smoke. What will you do? What can the problem be?

Solution

Tell the surgeon to remove the FIS cable and drapes quickly. Examine the patient for any evidence of burns on his skin.

Discussion

The case is similar to one previously reported (1). In that case, after it was ascertained that there was smoke present in the room, the light was turned on. Smoldering drapes over the pubes symphysis were readily seen where the FIS cable was lying on the drapes. The surgeon removed the FIS cable and the drapes were seen to stop smoking immediately. The patient was examined under the drapes and luckily no evidence of burns was found. He had an uneventful recovery. In another case report, the disconnected FIS cable ignited disposable, nonwoven paper surgical drapes that were trapped in an enriched pocket of oxygen. Oxygen had accumulated under the drapes from a faulty inflation connector of a pneumatic tourniquet. The resulting flash fire severely burned the patient's leg (2). Based on these reports, it is obvious that the FIS illumination end should never be disconnected from its scope. This will ensure that the extensive heat generated by the light does not cause fire. Combustion takes place when there is combustible material (in our case, paper drapes), supporting atmosphere (oxygen), and a source of ignition (in our case, the FIS). In a laboratory setting, the FIS can produce a smoldering fire on surgical drapes in as little as 7 s (1). It is interesting to note that despite the manufacturers of FISs warning that a disconnected, and therefore unprotected, FIS cable can ignite drapes and other operating room materials, very few surgeons seem aware of these dangers.

In another laboratory study, the presence of a Bair Hugger under a surgical drape, when exposed to an unprotected FIS, significantly accelerated the time to first smoke. Paradoxically, the presence of the Bair Hugger prevented damage to the patient's gown. The forced air prevented the inferior layer from coming into contact with the fiberoptic light source, thus protecting the underlying patient gown. In an actual surgical setting, it is likely that the Bair Hugger would offer some protection to the patient's skin, directly below the surgical drape (3).

Recommendation

The possibility of burns is ever present in the operating room and constitutes almost as much a risk to patients as to staff. Burns are essentially dependent on the energy delivered to a certain volume of tissue and the rate at which that energy can be dissipated. Burns are more likely when the blood supply to a body part is poor (4). Although operating room burns do occur, very few cases have been reported (4,5).

References

1. Eggen MA, Brock-Utne JG. Fiberoptic illumination systems can serve as a source of smoldering fires. J Clin Monit 1994;10:244–246.
2. The ECRI Institute. OR fires caused by fiberoptic illumination systems. Health Devices 1986;15:132.
3. Williams DM, Littwin S, Patterson AJ, Brock-Utne JG. Fiberoptic light source-induced surgical fires – the contribution of forced-air warming blankets. Acta Anaesthesiol Scand 2006;50(4):505–508.
4. Monks PS. Safe use of electronic medical equipment. Anesthesia 1971;26: 264–280.
5. Brock-Utne JG, Downing JW. Rectal burns after the use of an anal stainless steel electrode/transducer system for monitoring myoneural junction. Anesth Anal 1984;63;1139–1144.

8
Inguinal Hernia Repair in a Diabetic Patient

A 54-yr-old man is admitted for an inguinal hernia repair. He has been a type 1 diabetic for 18 years. Two years ago he developed end stage renal disease (ESRD), secondary to his diabetic kidney. He now requires daily peritoneal dialysis. The peritoneal fluid used consisted of a glucose-containing dialysis fluid in the daytime and an overnight dialysis fluid using one exchange of 2 liters peritoneal fluid containing icodextrin (7.5% wt/vol) (Extraneal; Baxter Healthcare, Castlebar, Ireland). Icodextrin is a cornstarch-derived glucose polymer. His insulin regimen consisted of Human Insulatard (Novo Nordisk) before bed and humalog (Lispro) before his main meals. On the morning (7:00 am) of his surgery, in the preoperative holding area, his capillary blood sugar value was 480 mg/dl. He had not taken any insulin for 12 h and had been non per os since midnight. The blood sugar test was done with an AccuChek Active (Roche, Mannheim, Germany). There were no ketones in the urine, and the patient claimed his blood sugar had, in the past 2 yr, been running higher. You speak to the surgeon and decide on monitored anesthesia care, which includes local anesthesia and sedation. You order 12 U of fast-acting insulin to be given IV stat (7:00 am). There is a delay in getting the patient to the operating room, but at 7:40 am you are given the go-ahead to pick up the patient. Much to your surprise, you find the patient somewhat incoherent and sweating. You take blood for blood glucose estimation while you call for 50% glucose. When the 50% glucose ampoule arrives, you don't wait for the blood sugar result, but give the patient 50 ml of 50% glucose IV with good effect. You are wondering how only 12 U of the above insulin could have caused this hypoglycemia. The nurse now tells you that the AccuChek shows blood glucose of 320 mg/dl. You realize something is not right when the venous blood glucose results come back as 2 mmol/liter (normal fasting levels, 3.33–6.60 mmol/liter). You ask the lab to run the venous blood glucose estimation again. You get the same result. However, the patient was obviously hypoglycemic. Why is there such a discrepancy between the two blood sugar estimations?

Solution

Several reports have alerted physicians to the potential interference of dialysis fluid containing 7.5% icodextrin, with some glucose reagent systems using a glucose dehydrogenase enzyme with coenzyme pyrroloquinoline-quinone (GDH-PQQ) (1–3). The glucose reagent systems in question are, beside the AccuCheck, the ExacTech (MediSense), Advantage (Roche), and Glucotrend (Roche). The test strip devices can overestimate the true capillary blood glucose readings, leading to erroneous diagnosis of hyperglycemia. If the patient is then treated with insulin, severe and potentially life-threatening hypoglycemia can ensue. In this case, had there been no delay going to the operating room, and had the patient been given a general anesthetic instead of monitored anesthesia care, there would have been no clinical warning of hypoglycemia. If the hypoglycemia had been left undiagnosed, it could have led to serious consequences.

Discussion

It is interesting to note that a full year before the FDA approved Extraneal in United States in 2002, this problem was highlighted in England (4). The reason for this interference is the fact that up to 40% of the indwelling icodextrin is systemically absorbed and metabolized by alpha-amylase into several oligosaccharides, including maltose, maltotriose, and maltotetrose. The metabolite concentration peaks at 12 h after infusion into the peritoneum, but remains in the circulation for 7 d.

Manufacturers of glucose test strips have reported interference with their test results when the patient has low hematocrit and/or high uric acid levels. These manufactures include BM Diagnostics, MediSense, Bayer Diagnostics, Roche Diagnostics, Lifescan, and Hypoguard.

Recommendation

Before you rely on handheld glucose monitors, you must be sure that the specific monitor is compatible with icodextrin-based peritoneal dialysis fluid (3). Furthermore, take particular note of the patient with a low hematocrit and/or high uric acid levels.

References

1. Disse E, Thivolet C. Hypoglycemic coma in a diabetic patient on peritoneal dialysis due to interference of icodextrin metabolites with capillary blood glucose measurements. Diabetes Care 2004;27;2279.

2. Moberly JB, Mujais S, Gehr T, et al. Pharmacokinetics of icodextrin in peritoneal dialysis patients. Kidney Int Suppl 2002;81:S23–S33.
3. Hoftman N. Interference between Extraneal Peritoneal Dialysis and the Accu-Chek blood glucose monitor. Anesthesiology 2005;102:871.
4. Mehmet S, Quan G, Thomas S, Goldsmith D. Important cause of hypoglycaemia in patients with diabetes on peritoneal dialysis. Diabetic Med 2001;18:679–682.

9
The Case of the "Hidden" IV

A 55-yr-old man is admitted for emergency laparatomy after a stab to his abdomen. He is hemodynamically stable. He has no history of note, except for a previous stab, again, to his abdomen. His previous anesthesia and surgery have been uneventful. He arrives in the operating room with a 20-gauge (G) IV in his hand, which is seen to work well. He does not like needles and, because he is considered stable, routine rapid sequence induction is initiated without any problems. After induction, a 14-G peripheral IV is placed in the right hand and attached to a Hotline Fluid Warmer (SIMS Level 1, Inc., Rockland, MA) for possible blood transfusion. A central vascular line is inserted into the right subclavian vein without any problems. The CVP is running well and you aspirate back blood easily from all lumens. At the surgeon's request, the left arm with the 20-G IV is tucked alongside the patient's body. The right hand, with the 14-G IV, is placed "out" at 90 degrees to his body. The surgery commences and repairs of both small and large intestines are needed. Four hours into the operation, the urine output decreases. The surgeon tells you there is no urine in the bladder. The central venous pressure (CVP), as measured with your triple-lumen IV set, is within normal limits. Through the 20-G IV (the IV is now seen to be working "great"), furosemide 10 mg is given and a dopamine drip is commenced. After 30–40 min, no improvement in urine output is seen. The patient is still cardiovascularly stable with a normal CVP, but the urine output has only been 3 ml in the last hour. You give more furosemide and increase your dose of dopamine again via your 20-G IV. However, 30 min later there is still no improvement in urine output. Before contemplating other drugs/doses/fluids what should you do?

Solution

Check your IV line. The problem in a previously reported case was that when we examined the 20-G IV from the IV bag to its insertion, we found that the IV line was cut 30 cm from where 20-G needles were placed in the vein (1). Interestingly, the distal end attached to the 20-G catheter had a tight knot, while the proximal end was completely open. It now became obvious why the IV was working "great." We could not ascertain how this happened, as all concerned denied any involvement. Somehow, the IV was cut and a knot was made either before or after the IV cut. It is of course possible that the tucking of the right arm with a sheet could have made a knot in the IV tubing and the surgeon later cut the IV proximately to the knot.

Discussion

In a previous publication, the problem with the "hidden" IV was highlighted (1). The term hidden IV is used when the surgeon requests one or both arms to be tucked beside the anesthetized patient's body during surgery. If the arm or arms have an IV in them, then the IV is hidden from view. Serious complications can arise when the IV insertion site is hidden. One of the more serious complications is large infiltration of fluids into the subcutaneous tissues of hand/arm/feet. I have seen a case where a right arm had to be amputated above the elbow following a 5-h cardiac bypass procedure, where liters of fluids and blood were pumped into the subcutaneous tissue of the forearm.

Recommendation

The message of this case is; if you have an IV that you can see is working, use it rather than an IV that is hidden. In this case, the use of the triple-lumen CVP line would have been perfect. The other point of this story is always worry about a hidden IV that suddenly starts to work great or suddenly does not work at all. Even if you are at risk of annoying the surgeon while checking your IV site, remember that you are looking after the patient. The fact that you may delay the surgeon for a minute or two is of no consequence.

Reference

1. Kim A, Brock-Utne JG. Another potential problem with the "hidden IV." Can J Anaesth 1998;45:495–496.

10
Postoperative Painful Eye

A 50-yr-old female, American Society of Anesthesiologists physical status 1, is scheduled for laparoscopic cholecystectomy. Her history is noncontributory. She takes no medication and has no allergies. The patient is otherwise healthy and has no complaints. She has removed her glasses and states that she does not use any contact lenses. You are joined by a medical student who put all the monitors on the patient, including the oxygen saturation monitor on her right index finger. The patient is induced, and the medical student ventilates the patient by mask. He places an endotracheal tube in the trachea successfully. The anesthetic proceeds uneventfully and she wakes up pain free and is taken to the recovery room in a stable condition. About 1 h later, the patient is still in the recovery room. You are called by the recovery room nurse to tell you that the patient is complaining of a painful eye. What will you do and what could the cause be?

Solution

You call for an ophthalmology consult. Corneal abrasion is suspected and the diagnosis confirmed by fluorescein staining. The treatment consists of eye ointment and taping the eye closed until resolution of the injury. The patient made an uneventful recovery.

Discussion

There are many causes of postoperative corneal abrasions. These have been highlighted by White and Cross in 1998 and include face masks, the anesthesiologist's hands, watch strap, or name badge, laryngoscopy during endotracheal intubation, surgical drapes and instruments, skin preparation solutions, or the direct irritant effect of inhalation anesthetic agents (1). In the postoperative period, the eye may be injured by facemasks, the patient's finger, or blankets or linen (1). The latter is especially true if the patient is in a lateral position (1). In this case, the cause of the corneal abrasion was most likely caused the disposable pulse oximeter probe, as all of the above causes could be excluded (2). The recovery nurse saw the patient rub her eye with the right index finger. This had the oximeter probe attached to it.

Recommendation

The ring finger may be a more appropriate site for the pulse oximeter, rather than the index finger. This avoids possible corneal abrasion when the patient rubs his/her eye in the immediate postoperative period (2,3).

References

1. White E, Crosse MM. The aetiology and prevention of peri-opeative corneal abrasions. Anaesthesia 1998;53:157–161.
2. Brock-Utne JG, Botz G, Jaffe RA. Perioperative corneal abrasions. Anesthesiology 1992;77:221.
3. Brock-Utne JG. The aetiology and prevention of peri-opeative corneal abrasion. Anaesthesia 1998;53:829.

11
Awake Craniotomy with Language Mapping

A 43-yr-old, 120 kg man, American Society of Anesthesiologists physical status 2, is being given local anesthesia with monitored anesthesia care (MAC) for an awake craniotomy. His history includes previous surgery under general anesthesia for resection of an astrocytoma. He presented with severe seizure disorder, mainly caused by further growth of the cerebral tumor. He is very nervous about having this procedure awake. Initially, remifentanil, and propofol infusion with local anesthesia provided adequate operating conditions. All sedation is turned off during the language mapping because the patient needs to be fully alert and cooperative. The patient is now only minimally sedated. Because his face is covered with drapes, he complains of severe claustrophobia and serious lack of air. His SpO_2 is 100%. Despite increasing the nasal oxygen to 10 liters/min and providing 15 liters/min of oxygen around his face from the absorber circuit of the Narcomed 2B anesthesia machine, no symptomatic relief is seen. Further sedation is not indicated because he needs to follow commands during the language mapping. His complaints are now becoming so serious that he wants the mapping and surgery stopped. Besides inducing general anesthesia, is there anything else that you could recommend?

Solution

In a previous case (1), we blew forced cold air (13.5°C) from a Polar Air Model 600 (Augustine Medical Corporation, Eden Prairie, MN) over the patient's face. This gave immediate relief from the feelings of lack of air and claustrophobia. The language mapping was completed successfully, and he made an uneventful recovery.

Discussion

Awake craniotomy without language mapping is relatively easy. With language mapping, it can be very challenging at best. Communication with the patient is of utmost importance during the procedure, so that the integrity of the speech center is maintained. The patient must understand, before surgery that he/she will have to lie still for hours in one position. Propofol and remifentanyl infusion has made this procedure well tolerated by most patients, but when it is turned off, problems can arise (2). Lack of air underneath the drapes can be very disturbing. We have several times used the Polar Air technique with good effect when the patient complains of claustrophobia and lack of air.

Recommendation

In awake craniotomy, remember to blow cold air over the patient's face, as this can often help to bring about a successful language mapping procedure.

References

1. Gerstner M, Eckinger P, Tew P, Brock-Utne JG. Another use of the "Bair Hugger." Can J Anaesth 1999;46:200.
2. McDougall RJ, Rosenfeld JV, Wrennall JA, Harvey AS. Awake craniotomy in an adolescent. Anaesth Intensive Care 2001;29:423–425.

12
Gum Elastic Bougie: Tips for Its Use

Today, you are working with a medical student in what would seem to be a straightforward surgical list. The first patient is a 40-yr-old female for a laparoscopic cholecystectomy. On examination, she has a class 2 airway, weighs 80 kg, and is 5'6". She has no other medical or surgical problems. The medical student places the IV and you induce anesthesia. The patient is easy to mask, and the medical student is doing a good job. You tell the medical student to get the laryngoscope out. He places the scope correctly, but tells you that he can't see anything. You look and have to agree with him. You decide the patient is a class 3. You take out your gum elastic bougie (GEB), also referred to as an endotracheal tube introducer, and place it blindly in what you think is the trachea. You pass a #7 endotracheal tube (ETT) over the GEB, but have difficulty advancing the ETT. You turn the ETT 90–180 degrees to the right and the ETT glides into what you think is the trachea. As you know, it is impossible to verify correct positioning without removing the GEB from the ETT. The medical student asks you, as you are about to remove the GEB, "Is there any way you could ascertain that you are in the trachea without removing the GEB from the ETT?" You remove the GEB and proceed to verify that the ETT is in the right place. You ponder the question and wonder if there is a way to do it. Is there?

Solution

The bronchoscopic swivel adaptor (PriMedico, Largo, FL) can be used to help confirm the correct placement of ETT without prior removal of the GEB (Fig. 12.1). This can be done by sliding the bronchoscopic swivel adaptor over the GEB via the bronchoscopic port. The bronchoscopic swivel adaptor is attached to the ETT, and correct placement can be confirmed by auscultation and capnography. The GEB can then be removed (1).

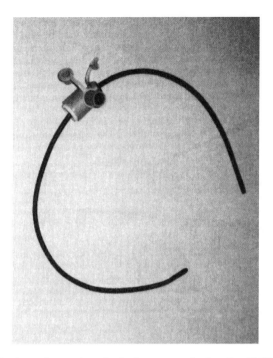

FIGURE 12.1. The bronchoscopic swivel adaptor attached to the GEB. (Reproduced with permission from Torralva PR, Macario A, Bruck-Utne JG. Anesth Analg 1999; 88:1187–1188.

Discussion

This technique can prove useful when using the GEB as a tube changer, allowing ventilation during the changeover, thereby minimizing the risk of hypoxia during this procedure (2).

The GEB was first described by Robert Macintosh in 1949 (3). Since then, it has proved its worth as a reliable and easy way to gain access to the difficult airway. However, like so many things, there is a little trick that one must know when using the GEB. If you encounter problems with passing the ETT over the GEB, then it is important to remember to turn the ETT either left or right 90–180 degrees before attempting to advance it. Under no circumstance should one force the GEB into the trachea or any other structures. If you feel you are in the trachea and, despite the aforementioned maneuver, you still do not succeed in advancing the ETT, then you should try a #6 ETT, which is the smallest ETT that an adult GEB will take. It is better to have a small tube than no tube at all.

Recommendation

The bronchoscopic swivel adaptor can be used to confirm the correct placement of the ETT without removing the GEB.

References

1. Torralva PR, Macario A, Brock-Utne JG. Another use of a bronchoscopic swivel adapter. Anesth Analg 1999;88:1187–1188.
2. Robles B, Hester J, Brock-Utne JG. Remember the gum-elastic bougie at extubation. J Clin Anesth 1993;5:329–331.
3. Macintosh RR. An aid to oral intubation. Br Med J 1949;1:28.

13
External Vaporizer Leak During Anesthesia

A 45-yr-old patient, American Society of Anesthesiologists physical status 2, is to undergo a removal of a cerebral tumor under general anesthesia. An anesthesia machine (Drager Fabius GS, Telford, PA) and breathing system check are performed before the patient's arrival. The Drager Vapor 2000 (Drager Medical AG, Lubeck, Germany) sevoflurane vaporizer is seen to be full. Noninvasive monitors are placed, and after preoxygenation the patient is anesthetized in a routine manner. Invasive monitors are placed and the operating table is turned 180 degrees from the anesthesia machine. The operation proceeds uneventfully until about 2 h into the case, when you suddenly smell anesthesia vapor around the anesthesia machine. You think you can smell more vapor around the vaporizer, but you are not sure. All vital signs are within normal limits. There are no warnings to indicate low minute volumes, apnea, or nonventilation of the patient. The rotameters show adequate flow and the pipeline pressure is 50 psi. The expired tidal volume is 600 ml, peak pressure is 25 cm and the respiratory rate is 8. End-tidal CO_2 and sevoflurane are within normal limits. (Datex Capnomac Ultima, Helsinki, Finland). What will you do? Will you ignore this finding or get another machine? Is there any way of identifying more precisely where the leak originates?

Solution

The best thing to do is to disconnect the CO_2/anesthetic agent sampling tube from the Datex Capnomac machine and use the sampling tube to "sniff" around the vaporizer and anesthesia machine. In this case, the cause of the smell was a leaking vaporizer.

Discussion

We have previously reported four different vaporizers of the Drager Vapor 2000 variety leaking vapor when in use (1). We believe that the problem with the above vaporizers is that they have been damaged during refilling.

When filling these vaporizers, the lever does not need to be flush with the front of the vaporizer. The lever should only be pushed to achieve slight resistance. Closing the lever all the way damages the filling port, and thereby causes a leak.

The "sniff" method was successful in identifying the leaks in all of the above vaporizers. We did not change the vaporizer until the end of the case. We were advised by our bioengineering technicians that this could not be done during the surgical operation. Because the amount of vapor that was leaking was minimal, we were not concerned. A bigger leak would have necessitated a machine change, or the use of another vaporizer on the existing machine.

The "sniff method" may also be used to identify small leaks in the anesthetic circuit, for example, a pinhole in the tubing from the ventilator to the sodalime absorber.

Recommendation

When you smell vapor around your anesthesia workstation or if you have a small leak in your circuit, don't forget the "sniff method."

Reference

1. Bolton P, Brock-Utne JG, Zumaran AA, Cummings J, Armstrong D. A simple method to identify an external vaporizer leak (the "Sniff" method). Anesth Analg 2005;101:606–607.

14
Manual Ventilation by a Single Operator: With Patient Turned 180 Degrees Away from the Anesthesia Machine

You are anesthetizing a healthy, American Society of Anesthesiologists physical status 1 young man for nasal reconstruction. He is taken to the operating room and routine monitors are placed. He is anesthetized, and the airway is secured uneventfully. He is disconnected from the ventilator and the table turned 180 degrees. The medical student who is working with you asks, "Why don't you turn the patient 180 degrees and then put him to sleep?" You explain that your arms are not long enough to hold the mask and the reservoir bag on the anesthetic machine. He sees your point. However, you wonder if there is a way to do this relatively safely with the existing equipment that you have available to you. Do you know a way?

Solution

It is called Omar's slave, and Dr. Omar was one of the best clinical anes-thesiologists I have ever had the pleasure to work with. He taught me this technique. Omar's slave (1) makes it possible for one operator to stand at the head of the table, 180 degrees away from the anesthesia machine, and control both the airway and manually ventilate the lungs. The modification consists of using a Portex straight gas sampling connection with a Luer port and cap (Sims Portex, Fort Meyers, Fl) and place it where the reservoir bag is situated on the anesthesia machine (North American Drager, Telford, PA). This sampling connection is then connected to 8–12-foot-long (22 mm diameter) anesthetic tubing. The other end of the anesthetic tubing is extended to the head of the operating table and fitted with a valve with a bleed vent from a Baby Safe Resuscitator (Vital Signs, Totowa, NJ) (Figs. 14.1 and 14.2).

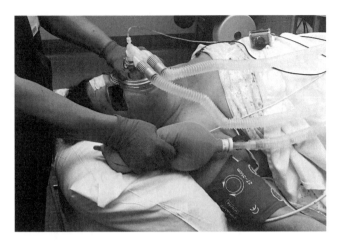

FIGURE 14.1. With the patient turned 180 degrees from the anesthesia machine, the anesthesiologist can ventilate the patient's lungs.

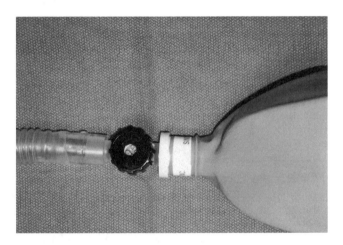

FIGURE 14.2. One end of the anesthetic tubing (not shown) is connected to the anesthesia machine where the reservoir bag is situated. The other end of the anesthetic tubing (shown in this figure) is connected to a Portex straight gas sampling connection. This, again, is connected to the valve assembly from Baby Safe Resuscitator including the reservoir bag (Vital Signs, Totowa, NJ). The whole length of the anesthetic tubing is 8–12 feet long.

Discussion

A study was undertaken (1) that showed that Omar's slave could function as intended. This technique is to be undertaken only by experienced anesthesiologists who have a surgeon and a nurse in the room, in case anything untoward should happen. Furthermore, Omar's slave must be checked for leaks and the patients must have class 1 or 2 airways and be of normal weight and height. I have personally used this in healthy patients on numerous occasions without any problems.

Recommendation

Omar's slave can be used by a single operator for manual ventilation of a patient turned 180 degrees from the anesthetic machine while maintaining minute ventilation and normal ETCO2.

Reference

1. Chu LF, Harrison K, Brock-Utne JG. Manual ventilation of a patient turned 180 degrees away from the anesthesia machine by a single operator. International Research SocAnnual meeting. New Orleans, LA. 21–23 March 2003.

15
Life-Threatening Arrhythmia in an Infant

A 5-mo-old child was scheduled for elective correction of transposition of the great arteries (Sennings procedure). She was diagnosed with the transposition immediately after birth, and a balloon septostomy was performed with good results. Before this proposed operation, the child was in good physical condition and weighed 5.9 kg. She tolerated the operation well and came off cardiopulmonary bypass uneventfully. She was paralyzed, ventilated, and sedated postoperatively. Her cardiovascular system was supported with small continuous doses of dopamine, phentolamine, and epinephrine with good effect. However, a persistent tachycardia ranging from 140 to 230 beats/min led to a decrease in mean arterial pressure and contributed to renal insufficiency with a rising creatinine. Peritoneal dialysis was initiated successfully. However, the tachyarrhythmia did not improve. Digoxin (Lanoxin) 0.16, 0.08, and 0.08 mg was given according to recommendation for children aged 2 wk–2 yr (0.04–0.06 mg/kg was given IV over the next few hours). However, no improvement was seen, and episodes of tachycardia up to 360 beats/min were seen even after the child was fully digitalized. Verapamil, propranolol, lidocarine, and phenytoin were given with no effect on this life-threatening arrhythmia. The patient was now completely anuric. An arterial blood gas showed pH 7.33, pCO_2 33 mmHg, BE 7.7 mmol/l, and pO_2 92 mmHg on FiO_2 0.4. The child had been in the intensive care unit (ICU) for over 24 h, and the fact that the serum potassium had risen to 5.9 mmol/liter caused great concern. The standard recommended treatment of high potassium, including normalizing the pH and giving glucose-insulin infusion, was started. The peritoneal dialysis fluid with potassium-free solutions was changed. Despite all this, a repeat potassium showed a further increase to 7.8 mmol/liter. Serum calcium and magnesium were within normal limits. The child was now critical, as besides the increased serum potassium and anuria, her cardiovascular system showed a heart rate of 300 beats/min and a mean arterial pressure of 48 mmHg. What was going wrong? Was there anything that could be done? If so, what?

Solution

This case is akin to a previously described case (1). The cause of the problem was digoxin intoxication, as the digoxin values came back at 8.1 nmol/liter (therapeutic range 1.2–2.5 nmol/liter). When this information became available, Fab (Digibind) was given IV in a recommended dose of 14.2 mg over a 60-s period. Within a minute after the administration of Fab, the tachyarrhythmia converted to a regular sinus rhythm at a rate of 140 beats/min. The mean arterial pressure increased from 48 to 65 mmHg. The need for inotropic, as well as ventilatory, support steadily decreased over a 24-h period. It is interesting to note that serum potassium normalized within 20 min after Fab was given. No adverse reactions were seen during and after the administration of Fab. The child was discharged from the ICU 3 d later and was doing very well.

Discussion

Recognition and treatment of digitalis toxicity is at times difficult. Mortality from digitalis overdoses varies, depending on numerous patient-specific factors, as well as the extent of toxicity (2). The cause of death in digitalis intoxication is mainly caused by fatal arrhythmias (3).

The patient described in the referenced case (1) showed an automatically accelerated atrioventricular (AV) junctional tachycardia, which is typically seen in acute digoxin overdose. Digoxin can produce many types of arrhythmias. They are mainly caused by depression or blockade of conduction and/or enhanced impulse formation. Enhanced impulse formation may appear in the form of atrial, junctional, or ventricular arrhythmias. Disturbances of conduction can occur in the sinus and AV nodes. Sinus bradycardia, sinus arrest, or sinoatrial block are common, and are caused by the interference of conduction in the sinus node. Depression of the AV node can present as second- or third-degree AV block. Early toxicity may present with prolongation of the PR interval. In a healthy heart, an acute overdose of digitalis leads to AV conduction disturbance with very few incidences of ventricular arrhythmias or ectopy (4,5). In contrast, the diseased heart frequently responds to an overdose with a lot of ectopic impulses, usually from a ventricular foci (5).

Hyperkalemia and refractory hypotension are common symptoms of digitalis toxicity, but are thought to be uncommon in children (2). In the case described, hypotension proved very difficult to treat with conventional inotropic support.

Hypoxemia, acidosis, hypokalemia, hypercalcemia, and hypomagnesemia may increase the irritability of the heart, resulting in arrhythmias. In our case, hypoxia, severe acidosis, hypokalemia, hypercalcemia, and hypomagnesemia were not present during and after the administration of digoxin.

Renal insufficiency can lead to hyperkalemia, however. In our case, the patient was receiving continuous peritoneal dialysis and laboratory values demonstrated stable values until the actual incident.

In the case described, there was a rapid increase in serum potassium approximately 28 h after full digitalization. This has been previously described (2,6). An increase in serum potassium in digitalis overdose has been suggested to be a prognostic sign to a poor outcome (7). In that report (7), the authors reported a mortality rate of 35% in patients who were treated conventionally for serum potassium greater than 5 mmol/liter. Fab has been shown to resolve ventricular and supraventricular extopy within 24 h and often within 4 hours in pediatric patients with digitalis intoxication (2). In our case, the rapid reversal of both cardiac and extracardiac manifestations of digoxin toxicity was unexpected, but nevertheless lifesaving.

Recommendation

The reader should note from this case that digoxin overdose can occur in infants, especially when renal impairment is present and despite reports that children seem to be less sensitive to the drug (3,8). Specific treatment with Fab should be considered, certainly when a refractory hyperkalemia occurs.

References

1. Husby P, Farstad M, Brock-Utne JG, et al. Immediate control of life-threatening digoxin intoxication in a child by use of digoxin-specific antibody fragments (Fab). Paediatr Anaesth 2003;13;541–546.
2. Woolf AD, Wenger TL, Smith TW, et al. Results of multicenter studies of digoxin-specific antibody fragments in managing digitalis intoxication in the pediatric population. Am J Emerg Med 1999;9:16–20.
3. Bayer MJ. Recognition and management of digitalis intoxication: implications for emergency medicine. Am J Emerg Med 1991;9:29–32.
4. Fowler RS, Rath L, Keith JD. Accidental digitalis intoxication in children. J Pediatr 1964;64:188–199.
5. Smith TW, Willerson JT. Suicidal and accidental digoxin ingestion. Circulation 1971;44:29–36.
6. Ooi H, Colucci WS. Pharmacological treatment of heart failure. In: Hardman JG, Limbird LE, Goodman Gilman A, eds. The Pharmacological Basis of Therapeutics. New York: McGraw-Hill Companies; 2001:901–932.
7. Gaultier M, Bismuth C. L'intoxcation digtalique aigue. La Rev d'Practicien 1978;28:4565–4579.
8. Hoffman BF, Bigger JT. Digitalis and allied cardiac glycosides. In: Goodman Gilman A, Rall TW, Nies AS, Taylor P, eds. The Pharmacological Basis of Therapeutics. New York: Pergamon Press; 1990:814–839.

16
Tongue Ring: Anesthetic Risks and Potential Complications

A 22-yr-old female, American Society of Anesthesiologists physical status 1, is scheduled for an elective diagnostic laparoscopy under general anesthesia. Her history is unremarkable. She takes no medication and she has no history of allergy. On the day of surgery, it is discovered the patient's tongue is pierced with a silver dumbbell-shaped piece of jewelry. This was not noticed by the preoperative clinic staff or mentioned in the surgeon's note. The jewelry is seen in the anterior one-third of her tongue and is sticking out of the tongue by 1 cm. You request that she remove the tongue ring, but she is reluctant to do so as it has been put in only 3 weeks ago. You warn her of the potential dangers, but she refuses to remove the tongue ring. You attempt to find a colleague that would be willing to do the case with the ring in situ. However, all your colleagues are either busy or reluctant to do the case. This leaves you with two options:

(A) Tell her that you would be happy to do the anesthetic if she removes the ring before surgery. If she refuses to remove the ring, you will cancel the case.
(B) Do the case with the ring in situ.

What will you do?

Solution

The answer is option A; just say no (1). Refuse to do the case with the ring in situ (2,3). Despite reports that patients have been anesthetized successfully with jewelry in situ, I would recommend that she take the ring out.

Discussion

There are two major concerns with jewelry worn by the patient in the operating room. One is burns; rings or needles (4) and metals (5) can be a source of "alternate-site burn." This is especially true for the older models of ground-referenced generators. Newer electrosurgical generators are designed to avoid alternate burn sites. However, in the instruction for use of these newer generators, it states clearly, "Patient safety is the highest concern, and one is not well served when jewelry is present in the patient undergoing surgery when electrosurgical generators are used." The insert goes on to say that if the jewelry is not removed the RISK ASSOCIATED WITH THE PRESENCE OF JEWELRY MUST BE ASSUMED BY THE PATIENT AND THE HOSPITAL. As Rosenberg et al. (1) state: "If the companies that produce the equipment are against wearing jewelry and are willing to place the responsibility on us, why should we condone wearing rings in the operating room?" I agree.

The other concern: if a tongue ring is left in situ for the operation, the ring may cause pressure necrosis to the tongue. The ring may also become dislodged and fall into the trachea.

Mandabach et al. (2) have argued that one should evaluate the decision to cancel or not to cancel these cases on a case-by-case basis. He suggests the following precautions. First, jewelry is removed if possible. Second, the dispersive plate is placed as far away as possible from the surgical field. Third, electrocautery is not used if the jewelry is close to the site of surgery. Fourth, the surgeon should use a bipolar electrosurgical unit. This utilizes less power because the current passes only between the tips of the unit unlike the monopolar unit, where the current passes from the tip throughout the body on its way to the dispersive pad (6). Fifth, use the newer electrosurgical units with isolated generators that limit the risks of alternate burning sites. The word here is LIMIT. I leave it to the reader to decide, but I would just say NO.

Recommendation

When faced with this sort of problem, I believe that you must be firm and say no for all the reasons mentioned, and not least for the potential medical legal ramifications. To leave the ring in could cause harm, and you do not want to do that.

References

1. Rosenberg AD, Young M, Berstein RL, Albert DB. Tongue Rings: Just say NO. Anesthesiology 1998;89:1279.
2. Oyos TL. Intubation sequence for patient presenting with tongue ring. Anesthesiology 1998;88;279.
3. Mandabach MG, McCann DA, Thompson GE. Body art: Another concern for the anesthesiologist. Anesthesiology 1998;88:279–280.
4. Rappaport W, Thompson S, Wong R, Leong S, Villar H. Complications associated with needle localization biopsy of the breast. Surg Gynecol Obstet 1991; 171:303–306.

5. Brock-Utne JG, Downing JW. Rectal burn after the use of an anal stainless steel electrode/transducer system for monitoring myoneural junction. Anesth Analg 1984;63:1141–1142.
6. Ehrenwerth J. Electrical safety. In: Barash PG, Cullen BF, Stoelting RK, eds. Clinical Anesthesia. 3rd ed. Philadelphia: Lippincott-Raven Publishers; 1996: 137–559.

17
Hasty C-Arm Positioning: A Recipe for Disaster

You have anesthetized an otherwise healthy man for a neurosurgical procedure. He is 54-yr-old, weighs 110 kg, and is 6 feet tall. He is placed in a left lateral position. The surgeon is in a bit of a rush, and before the patient is appropriately secured, the surgeon moves the C-arm into position over the operating room (OR) table (Skyton 3; John Cudia & Assoc., Morgan Hill, CA). Suddenly, the table goes into a full left-lateral tilt without anyone touching the table control situated at the head of the table. You grab the patient's head and the endotracheal tube and call for help. The surgeon and nurses, with outstretched hands, are preventing the patient from hitting the floor. They call for a gurney, and as you await its arrival the table is still moving in a full left-lateral tilt. What will you do?

Solution

This case is akin to one previously described (1). In that case, we held the patient's head and the endotracheal tube. What saved the day was unplugging the OR table from its electrical outlet. The table stops abruptly with a tilt of 30–40 degrees to the floor. His gurney was quickly brought back into the room, and the anesthetized patient was safely transferred to the gurney. With the patient safe, we searched for a possible cause and found that the bottom end of the C-arm (i.e., the part of the C-arm that is closest to the floor) was wedged onto the floor control of the Skyton OR table. The C-arm was removed, and the OR table was again plugged into the electrical outlet. The OR table control was now able to function correctly, and the patient was placed back on the operating table. The surgery was completed uneventfully.

Discussion

It is important to remember that the patient must be secured as soon as the positioning is complete. Regarding the patient described above he would most likely have fallen on the floor despite having been secured. This is because there was and is usually only one strap (over the thighs) that keeps the patient on the OR table. In all cases where strange and bizarre things happen in the OR, the patient's safety and welfare is of paramount importance. I remember having a 140 kg, 5′4″ inch woman anesthetized in the lithotomy position for a gynecological surgical procedure. When the surgeon ordered more Trendelenburg, the patient started to slide headfirst off the table. There was no time to get the OR table control to reverse the Trendelenburg, as she was gathering speed. I tried to hold her, but was unsuccessful. She kept gliding off the table, headfirst. The surgeon shouted, "What are you doing?" I called for help, but no one came in time, so I grabbed the head with one arm and the endotracheal tube with the other hand. She kept sliding, and to prevent her head from hitting the floor, I sat down on the floor and her head landed in my lap. Eventually help arrived, the Trendelenburg was reversed, the patient was repositioned on the OR table, and the surgery completed. The cause of this mishap was that the patient's short, large legs were inadequately secured into the stirrups. Everything went well, except that unbeknown to everyone, a lap was left behind in her peritoneal cavity. Another operation had to be performed to remove it. The patient was reportedly happy, as she thought she had malignant tumor in her abdomen after the first operation and was ecstatic when she was told it was only a lap left behind from the previous surgery. It is important to realize that in cases where the legs cannot be secured adequately in the stirrups, Trendelenburg must be limited.

A C-arm has been known to be activated unintentionally, thereby pressing the head of an anesthesiologist toward the patient's head as he was busy securing the airway (2).

Accidental activation of control knobs on an x-ray table has also been reported to trap an anesthesiologist between the wall and the x-ray table, leaving him unable to move and too close to the anesthetized patient under his care (3).

Recommendation

Beware of a hasty surgeon working a C-arm before the patient is secured onto the OR table, and make sure the OR table floor control is far away from the bottom part of the C- arm.

References

1. Bolton P, Zisook G, Brock-Utne JG. Hasty C-arm positioning: a recipe for disaster. Anesth Analg 2002;102:644.
2. Riley RH, Coombs LJ. X-ray machine assaults anaesthetist. Med J Australia 2006;182:368.
3. Riley RH. Anchoring an anaesthetist. Med J Australia 2002;177:687–688.

18
Inability to Remove a Nasogastric Tube

A 4-wk-old, American Society of Anesthesiologists physical status 1 boy is scheduled for a pyloromyotomy. Before anesthesia, his nasogastric tube (NG) is removed. The anesthesia induction and maintenance is uneventful. A new NG is inserted easily during surgery (Argyle feeding tube, size Ch 8, external diameter 2.7 mm × 107 cm; Sherwood Medical, St. Louis, MO). Its correct position is verified by air insufflations and slight dilation of the stomach. The patient is taken to the pediatric intensive care unit for recovery. Several hours later, the nurse attempts to manipulate the NG because it seems to be occluded. While she is attempting to move the NG, she is surprised to see a loop of the NG suddenly appear in the mouth. She pushes the NG in again but after that she cannot move the NG up or down. You are called and confirm that the NG is stuck. What will you do?

Solution

Examine with your finger the baby's mouth to ascertain if the NG has curled up in the back of the pharynx. You feel the NG, but you have difficulty ascertaining what is going on. You call for fluoroscopy and find that the NG has formed a knot with a large loop at the level of the oropharynx. You cut the NG as it emerges from the nostril. Under brief sedation with propofol, you retrieve the NG orally with a Magill forceps, using your laryngoscope under direct visual control. You then reinsert a new NG under fluoroscopic control.

Discussion

This case is similar to one previously reported (1). In that case, it was hypothesized that the NG was initially inserted too far. This allowed the NG to form a loop in the oropharynx. It is possible that, with the nurse manipulating the NG, a knot with a large loop was formed. This loop prevented the NG from being removed via the nose. If blind traction had been used to remove the NG, the baby would have suffered severe damage to its palate.

Similiar cases of inability to remove a nasogastric tube can be seen in other cases (2–8).

Recommendation

If a NG cannot be removed easily, an x-ray should be done. Always check the markings on the inserted NG (if present) to make sure it is not inserted too far.

References

1. Michel Ives, Veyckemans F, Van Boven M. Unusual Complication of a nasogastric tube insertion. Anesth Analg 1997;84:471.
2. Hefner CD, Wylie JH, Brush BF. Complications of gastrointestinal intubation. Arch Surg 1961;83:163–76.
3. Dees G. Difficult nasogastric tube insertions. Emerg Med Clin N Am 1989;7:177–182.
4. Patow CA, Pruet CW, Fetter TW, Rosenberg SA. Nasogastric tube perforation of the nasopharynx. South Med J 1985;78:1362–1365.
5. Lind LJ, Wallace DH. Submucosal passage of a nasogastric tube complicating attempted intubation during anesthesia. Anesthesiology 1978;49:145–147.
6. Dorsey M, Schwinder L, Benemof JL. Unintentional endotracheal extubation by orogastric tube removal. Anesth Rev 1988;15:30–33.
7. Pousman RM, Koch SM. Endotracheal tube obstruction after orogastric tube placement. Anesthesiology 1997;87:1247–1248.
8. Au-Truong X, Lopez G, Joseph NJ, Ramez Salem M. A case of a nasogastric tube knotting around a tracheal tube: detection and management. Anesth Analg 1999;89:1583–1584.

19
An Unusual Cause of Difficult Tracheal Intubation

A 45-yr-old, 80 kg Sikh man from India is admitted for repair of scapholunate dislocation. His past medical history and physical exam is unremarkable. He is classified as American Society of Anesthesiologists physical status 1. He has a full beard and speaks English very well. He requests a regional block, but unfortunately it proves to be inadequate for the surgery. General anesthesia is decided upon. After preoxygenation, general anesthesia is induced with intravenous thiopental 250 mg, followed by succinylcholine 120 mg. Ventilation is easily accomplished by mask. At laryngoscopy, the patient's jaw is found not to be relaxed. Trismus is considered. The nerve stimulator shows loss of twitch. A Macintosh #3 laryngoscope blade is passed into the pharynx with great difficulty caused by the very restricted mouth opening. Only the epiglottis is seen, but you manage to successfully place a #7 endotracheal tube in the trachea.

He does not have a wired jaw nor does he have bilateral temporalmandibular joint disease. Why can he not open his mouth?

Solution

Further examination of his airway reveals the cause of the problem. His religious belief prevents him from cutting his hair. The excess hair has been put up in a bun on top of his head. From this bun, a long strand of hair is woven tightly together into a cord (0.5–1 cm wide) that goes under his jaw (Fig. 19.1). This cord is severely restricting the mouth opening.

Discussion

The above case is similar to two previous ones that describe this potential problem (1,2). In our case (1), our cursory preoperative examination did not reveal any airway abnormalities caused by disease or trauma to neck and/or jaw. Had we asked him to open his mouth, we would have discovered the patient's inability to do so. In another communication, we recommend that all bearded Sikhs should be examined preoperatively for beard

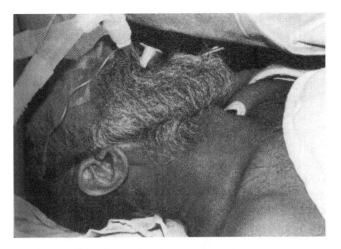

FIGURE 19.1. A bearded Sikh with a cord that severely restricts the mouth opening. With permission from Brodsky et al., 1991.

restrainers (3). We also recommend that the patient be informed that the cord may have to be loosened or even cut (3). However, Bhogal (4) disagrees strongly with cutting the cord as this is considered a serious religious sin. The interesting thing about this cord is that it can be made of any material. It can be elastic and therefore may have some give in it. The position of the bun can be placed anywhere on the top of the head. It can be nearer the forehead or nearer the occiput. The cord, which is attached to bun, can therefore be anywhere. If you know a Sikh is using the cord to restrain his beard, then you can ask him to manipulate the bun to make the cord looser or, better still, not to use the cord on the day of surgery. There is no religious objection to the latter.

Recommendation

A bearded Sikh will not object to not wearing the cord on the day of surgery. To have to cut it because you are unable to control his airway will be considered a serious sin by the patient.

References

1. Brodsky JB, Brock-Utne JG, Haddow GR, Azar DR. A hairy problem. Anesth Analg 1991;72:839.
2. Bhogal HS, Gan TJ. Awareness of Sikh custom of restraining a beard with a cord leading to possible airway problems. Anesth Analg 1999;1586.
3. Brock-Utne JG, Brodsky JB, Haddow GR. Bearded Sikhs and tracheal intubation Anesth Analg 2000;90:494.
4. Bhogal HS. Bearded Sikhs and tracheal intubation. Anesth Analg 2000;90:494.

20
Pulmonary Edema After Abdominal Laparoscopy

A 69-yr-old, 50 kg woman with pelvic pain is admitted for laparoscopic carbon dioxide laser lysis of pelvic adhesions. Her history for hypertension and hyperlipidemia is significant. Her clinical exam is unremarkable, and although there are no cardiac symptoms, her preoperative electro-cardiogram (ECG) shows a left anterior fascicular block. Her medication includes hydrochlorothiazide, triamterene, and gemfibrozil. She is not allergic to any medication. She is sedated with midazolam 2 mg IV and taken to the operating room. Thereafter, monitors are placed, and she has a successful induction of general endotracheal anesthesia. She is maintained with desflurane/fentanyl/oxygen/air mixture. Pancuronium is used for muscle relaxation. During the operation, the patient receives a total of 2,100 ml of crystalloid fluid IV over the 185-min procedure. (1,000 ml lactate Ringer's solution before the procedure started, 1,000 ml 0.9% saline during the first 90 min, and 100 ml 0.9% saline during the final 95 min). The surgeon infuses a lactated Ringer's solution through the laparoscope to wash away blood and debris and thereby improve vis-ualization. The nurse tells you that a total amount of 4,400 ml was instilled, and a similar amount was recovered by the surgeon while sucking out the peritoneal cavity. Her urinary output is 300 ml. At the end of the surgery, the neuromuscular blockade is reversed with glycopyrrolate and neo-stigmine. Spontaneous breathing ensues. The patient responds to verbal command and maintains a 10-s head lift. The endotracheal tube is removed, but, while still in the operating room, she becomes less alert and seems to have difficulty breathing. You give her 100% oxygen via mask and the saturation improves to 93% from 84%. Your nerve stimulator shows four strong twitches. Pupils are small to midsize, but you elect to give naloxone IV up to 0.4 mg. As expected, there is no clinical improvement. You examine the patient's chest and bilateral rales are heard over the lower half of her lung fields. You take her to the postoperative recovery ward and a chest x-ray confirms the diagnosis of pulmonary edema. How will you treat this? What investigations will you do? Why is the patient in pulmonary edema?

Solution

In this case, after asking the nurse again, the anesthesia team discovered that the amount of recovered fluid from the peritoneal cavity was only 1,950 ml compared to the 4,400 ml injected. It is the anesthesiologist's responsibility to ascertain what these numbers are at the end of the case. Do not rely on others for that information; check it yourself. Furosemide, 20 mg IV improved the patient over a 20–30 min period after a massive diuresis. It is advisable to do electrolyte estimations and an ECG. If the ECG shows new evidence of ischemia, the patient should be admitted for observation and serial cardiac enzymes should be done. In the previously described case, the patient was discharged from the hospital the following day and had an otherwise uneventful recovery (1).

Discussion

This patient was fine during general anesthesia because positive ventilation of the lung prevented any signs of excessive systemic fluid absorption. This case is akin to a previously reported case (1). It illustrates the fact that endoscopic procedures are not without significant anesthetic problems. One such complication is an excessive increase in intravascular volume resulting from absorption of irrigating fluid. This occurs in 0.14–0.34% of patients undergoing endoscopic uterine surgery (2). Excessive intravascular volume manifesting as hemolysis, hyponatremia, and mild disseminated intravascular coagulation and/or pulmonary edema has been reported with glycine (3), dextrose (4), sterile water (5), or dextran 70 (6) when these agents are used as the irrigating solutions. The factors that influence the degree of fluid absorption include injection pressure, extent of tissue trauma, and amount of fluid and duration of infusion.

This case shows that the aforementioned complications can also occur during nonuterine endoscopic surgery when crystalloid solution is used as irrigating fluid. It is important to realize that these patients undergo extensive preoperative bowel preparation. Therefore, their intravascular volume is depleted and, often, aggressive preoperative and/or intraoperative fluid resuscitation must be done. In this case, the fluid management was made even more problematic as she was on preoperative diuretic therapy for chronic hypertension.

Recommendation

In these cases, the amount instilled into the peritoneal cavity and the amount removed should be recorded every 15 min (1). Serum sodium levels should be checked when fluid absorption exceeds 1,500 ml (3). Had the patient not responded so quickly to the therapy, consideration as to placing a central line could be made. The same argument could be made for high-risk patients undergoing this procedure (1). It is the anesthesiologist's responsibility to ascertain the amount of fluid injected into, and the amount of fluid recovered from, the peritoneal cavity. Ideally, they should be equal.

References

1. Healzer JM, Nezhat C, Brodsky JB, Brock-Utne JG, Seidman DS. Pulmonary edema after absorbing crystalloid irrigating fluid during laparoscopy. Anesth Analg 1994;78:1207.
2. Hulka JF, Peterson HB, Phillips JM, Surrey MW. Operative hysteroscopy. American Association of Gynecologic Laparoscopists 1991 membership survey. J Reprod Med 1993;38:572–573.
3. van Boven MJ, Singelyn F, Donnez J, Gribomont BF. Dilutional hyponatremia associated with intrauterine endoscopic laser surgery. Anesthesiology 1989; 71:449–450.
4. Carson SA, Hubert GD Schriock ED, Buster JE. Hyperglycemia and hyponatremia during operative hysteroscopy with 50% dextrose. Fertil Steril 1989; 51:341–343.
5. D'Agosto J, Ali NMK, Maier D. Absorption of irrigating solutions during hysteroscopy: hysteroscopy syndrome. Anesthesiology 1990;72:379–380.
6. Mangar D. Anaesthetic implications of 32% dextran-70 (Hyskon) during hysteroscopy: hysteroscopy syndrome. Can J Anaesth 1992;39:975–979.

21
Difficult Laryngeal Mask Airway Placement: A Possible Solution

A 40-yr-old American Society of Anesthesiologists physical status 1 female with a Mallampati class 2 airway is scheduled for cystoscopy and biopsy of the bladder under general anesthesia. She weighs 80 kg and is 165 cm in height. Her only complaint is hematuria. This is her first hospital admission and first general anesthetic. She refuses a spinal or epidural. You induce general anesthesia with propofol 150 mg. The placement of the laryngeal mask airway (LMA) with the Brain technique proves impossible, as the LMA will not pass the junction with the posterior pharynx. You attempt to insert the LMA with other different techniques, including rotating the LMA 180 degrees, to no avail. Do you know of another technique using a stylet to insert the LMA?

Solution

Yodfat (1) was the first to describe a technique for LMA placement using a stylet. His method, which we have slightly modified, is described in the following paragraph (2).

A conventional endotracheal tube style (Slick Stylette; Polamedco, Marina del Rey, CA) is folded in half. This reduces its length to approximately 22 cm. The stylet is lubricated and inserted into the LMA to be used. Care must be taken to ensure that the tips of the stylet do not protrude beyond the LMA aperture bars. With the stylet in place in the LMA, the LMA is bent to 90 degrees, close to the junction of the airway tube and mask. The LMA is then lubricated in the usual manner. The LMA cuff is partially inflated, and the tip is curled anteriorly. The patient's mouth is opened by grasping the mandible with the nondominant hand while the LMA is inserted in a manner that effectively mimics the force vectors used in the Brain technique (Fig. 21.1). The tip of the LMA is placed against the hard palate and advanced using continuous pressure, rotating the LMA so that the mask follows the curvature of the airway into its final resting position in the pharynx. The strongly curved stylet serves as a functional

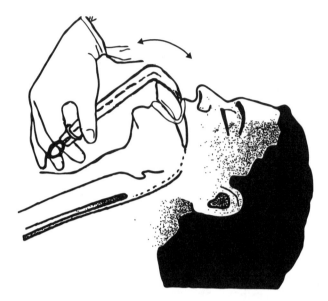

FIGURE 21.1. The LMA with stylet in place is inserted into the airway in a manner that mimics the original Brain technique. The figure has been simplified by omitting the nondominant hand, which would be used to grasp and lift the mandible. Reproduced with permission from Jaffe RA and Brock-Utne JG, 2002.

replacement for the operator's finger, the advantage being that it can be kept safely outside the patient's mouth. The stylet is then removed by withdrawing it from the LMA tube. Finally, the mask is inflated in the usual fashion.

Discussion

There is no doubt the Brain technique has been associated with less than satisfactory seating of the LMA. Brain insists that this is because many anesthesiologists do not use his technique correctly (4). Whatever the reason for the less than satisfactory result in placing the LMA, many use the half-twist or full-twist, 180-degree insertion technique. The original Brain technique describes the LMA as being held as a pen, with the index finger positioned against the proximal cuff. Then, with continuous pressure against the hard palate, the LMA is advanced into the pharynx. The main disadvantage of this technique is that the anesthesiologist's finger and knuckles may scrape against the patient's teeth. Patients with small mouth openings or difficult oropharyngeal passageways may require considerable effort, with multiple attempts to achieve proper LMA placement. Even in patients with normal airways, an anesthesiologist who is not blessed with slim fingers may get scraped by the patient's teeth.

Recommendation

It is worth practicing this modification of the Yodfat LMA insertion technique until it is done easily. When faced with a difficult LMA placement, this technique can prove to be of real benefit.

References

1. Yodfat US. Modified technique for laryngeal mask airway insertion. Anesth Analg 1999; 89:1327.
2. Jaffe RJ, Brock-Utne JG. A modification of the Yodfat laryngeal mask airway insertion technique. J Clin Anesth 2002;14:462–463.
3. Brimacombe J, Berry A. Insertion of the laryngeal mask airway – a prospective study of four techniques. Anesth Intensive Care 1992;21:89–92.
4. Brain AIJ. The Intavent laryngeal mask instruction manual. 2nd ed. Berkshire, UK: Brian Medical, Ltd.; 1991.

22
Postoperative Airway Complication After Sinus Surgery

A 28-yr-old man (American Society of Anesthesiologists physical status 1) with chronic sinusitis is scheduled for functional endoscopic sinus surgery (FESS). He has failed medical management. He is 84 kg and 5′10″ tall. He has had one previous general anesthetic for an acute appendix at age 10. Otherwise, his medical history and physical exam is unremarkable. He is presently not taking any medication and has no known allergies to medicines. He has a normal white cell count and his Hb is 14 mg%. After sedation with midazolam 2 mg IV, he is taken to the operating room, where a routine general anesthetic is induced uneventfully. Tracheal intubation (grade 1 view) is done atraumatically on the first attempt after ensuring that the patient is fully paralyzed with a nerve stimulator (vecuronium 7 mg). The pharynx is deemed normal both preoperatively and during endotracheal intubation. The endotracheal tube (ETT) is secured and bilateral air entry is recorded with the presence of CO_2 on the capnograph. General anesthesia is maintained with oxygen, nitrous oxide, isoflurane, morphine, and fentanyl. The operation lasts 90 min, and the vital signs throughout the surgery are within normal limits. The estimated blood loss is 900 ml. No airways or oral packs are used during the surgery, except for a nasal posterior pack that was placed before the FESS commenced and removed after surgery. The inferior nasal vault was not packed, but small hemostati sponges were placed in the ethmoid cavities. Before the patient fully awoke, the pharynx was gently suctioned using a Yankauer suction and an oral-gastric tube placed on its first attempt. Suction was applied, and the tube was withdrawn completely. With the patient fully awake and able to follow commands, the ETT is removed. Initially, in the recovery room, the patient is comfortable with stable vital signs. However, within 10 min he complains of difficulty in breathing. Despite supplemental oxygen (6 l/min) via an oxygen mask, his oxygen saturation decreased to 86%. You are called back, and when you examine the patient's chest you can hear only minimal scattered expiratory noises (stridors). Racemic epinephrine is given with minimal improvement. You put another saturation monitor on his finger but the saturation is still 86%. What will you do now?

Solution

Always remember to examine the throat, too. In this case, a large, swollen, and elongated uvula was seen. The tip of the uvula, deemed to be 13–14 cm long, could not be seen. The uvula, from time to time, triggered a gag reflex with coughing. In a previously reported similar case, dexamethsone 8 mg was administered and the nebulized racemic epinephrine continued (1). The head of the bed was elevated to 75 degrees. After 2 h, the patient was discharged from the recovery room to the ward. Dexamethazone (8 mg every 8 h) was continued. He was discharged home the next day with marked reduction in uvular swelling. There was no evidence of edema on postoperative day 3.

Discussion

There are many causes of uvulitis. The main causes include mechanical and thermal trauma, infection, chemical, an allergic reaction, and nonallergic complement-mediated disorders (2–6). From these references, the disconcerting fact is that uvular edema can develop any time from 45 min to 24 h after the event that caused it. Dexamethazone is considered the treatment of choice for uvular edema. This is caused by the drug's antiinflammatory potency, which is 25 times greater than that of hydrocortisone, and a long half-life of 36–72 h. Steroids exhibit their effects by decreasing capillary endotracheal permeability, leading to a decrease in mucosal edema, and by decreasing the inflammatory reaction by stabilizing lysosomal membranes. In posttraumatic uvulitis, steroids have been shown to bring about dramatic relief (7). If it is believed that the uvular edema is an allergic reaction, then diphenhydramine is recommended (2,6).

After this type of surgery, if you question a patient who complains of difficulty breathing, it is most likely that he/she will report that there is something lodged at the back of the throat. Besides the uvular edema, remember to look for other problems in the back of the pharynx, like dislodged packs or sponges, bone fragments, blood clots, or foreign bodies.

Recommendation

1. Always examine your patient's throat before anesthesia.
2. Should postoperative respiratory obstruction occur, always remember to examine the throat, not just the chest.
3. Uvular edema can be delayed for hours. It can also get worse before it gets better.
4. Treatment must be aggressive and the patient admitted to ICU.

References

1. Holden JP, Vaughan WC, Brock-Utne JG. Airway complication following functional endoscopic sinus surgery. J Clin Anesthesia 2002;14:154–157.
2. Haselby KA, McNiece WL. Respiratory obstruction from uvular edema in a pediatric patient. Anesth Analg 1982;65:1127–1128.
3. Mallat AM, Roberson J, Brock-Utne JG. Preoperative marijuana inhalation – an airway concern. Can J Anaesth 1996;43:691–693.
4. Shulman MS. Uvular edema without endotracheal intubation. Anesthesiology 1981;55:82–83.
5. Ravindran R, Priddy S. Uvular edema, a rare complication of endotracheal intubation. Anesthesiology 1978:48:374.
6. Seigne TD, Felske A, DelGiudice PA. Uvular edema. Anesthesiology 1978;49:375–376.
7. Hawkins DB, Crockett DM, Shum TK. Corticosteroids in airway management. Otolaryn Head Neck Surg 1983;91:593–596.

23
Investigating an Unusual Capnograph Tracing: Check Your Connections

You have anesthetized a healthy 24-yr-old man (American Society of Anesthesiologists physical status 1E) for an acute laparoscopic appendectomy. He has no history of previous anesthetic, he does not take medication regularly, and he has no history of allergy to medication. There is no family history of any problems with anesthesia. He is 75 kg and 6′0″ tall. After rapid sequence induction, you secure the airway and see a CO_2 wave form on the capnograph (Datex Capnomac Ultima; Datex, Helsinki, Finland; incorporates a sidestream CO_2 monitor), confirming bilateral air entry. The endotracheal tube is taped at 23 cm. The vital signs are normal. However, on closer inspection of the capnograph waveform, you now notice that the capnograph is very different than what you normally see (Fig. 23.1). The tracing starts from a zero and a normal plateau is reached, but just before the trace should normally go to zero, there is a marked peak in the tracing before rapidly returning to zero. Tidal volumes, respiratory rates, and minute volume are within normal limits. The peak pressure is 24 cm. The patient's vital signs remain normal. You have not seen anything like this before, and because you checked the Narcomed 2B (North America Dräger) anesthesia machine before administering the anesthetic, you are now wondering what this trace could mean. Should you be concerned? What do you think the problem is? What, if anything, can you do?

Solution

The cause of the problem is that the capnograph tubing from the patient's breathing circuit at the mouth end is not screwed in properly to the Datex capnograph aspirating port (1). As the Datex does not discriminate as to what gas is absorbed into the machine, room air is entrained and mixed with the patient's respiratory gases. Initially, this mixing gives a lower than normal plateau. However, the reason for the peak is that it corresponds to the inspiratory cycle of the ventilator. Mixed expired gases are forced up the capnograph tube during the initiation of inspiration, preventing less

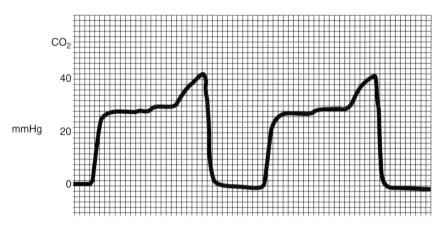

FIGURE 23.1. Capnograph wave form. (Reproduced with permission from Sims C. Anaesth Intens Care 1990;18:272.)

or no room air entrainment. These lead to the peak that is seen in the capnograph tracing.

Discussion

This unusual capnogram was a concern until the cause was found and easily rectified. The same size leak at the patient end of the sampling tube does not have as marked an effect (2). The described pattern is not seen when the patient is breathing spontaneously, but a false low–end-tidal CO_2

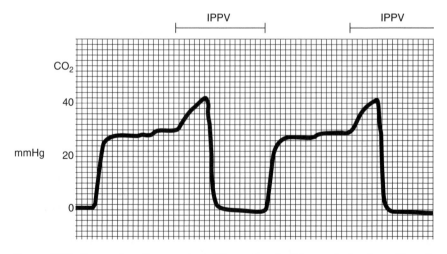

FIGURE 23.2. For explanation, see text. (Reproduced with permission from Sims C. Anaesth Intens Care 1990;18:272.)

measurement is seen with no terminal hump (2). During calibration, a falsely low–end-tidal CO_2 can be seen, and entrainment is present (2). This problem with the side stream carbon dioxide analysis cannot be seen with the mainstream carbon dioxide analyzer.

Capnography is the graphic display of CO_2 partial pressure in a "wave form" format. (Fig. 23.2) Capnography is superior to capnometry, which is the measurement of numerical display of CO_2 concentration on partial pressure in the patient's airway during the respiratory cycle. Capnography assesses not only alveolar ventilation, but the integrity of the airway, proper functioning of anesthesia delivery system, ventilator function, cardio-pulmonary function, and potential rebreathing. Capnography has been used, among other things, to diagnose incompetent and/or expiratory values (3), spontaneous respiratory effect, lung disease, and CO_2-absorbent exhaustion (4).

Recommendation

Capnography serves as an anesthesia disaster early warning system. Changes from a normal waveform must always be investigated and corrected if possible. In this case, the unusual waveform was caused by simple equipment failure.

References

1. Sims C. An unusual capnogram. Anaesth Intens Care 1990;18:272.
2. Prevedoros HP, Morris RW. An interesting capnograph tracing. Anaesth Intens Care 1990;18:271.
3. Gravenstein N. Manual of Complications During Anesthesia. JB Lippincott Co.; 1990.
4. Pond D, Jaffe RA, Brock-Utne JG. Failure to detect CO_2 absorbent exhaustion. Seeing is believing. Anesthesiology 2000;92:1196–1198.

24
A Respiratory Dilemma During a Transjugular Intrahepatic Portosystemic Shunt Procedure

A 54-yr-old, 55 kg man with a history of alcohol abuse and hepatitis is scheduled for a transjugular intrahepatic portosystemic shunt (TIPS). He has received sclerotherapy for variceal bleeding, but recurrent bleeding has ensued. He has no other major complaints. His international normalized ratio is 1.1. A radial arterial line is placed preoperatively together with a 16-gauge IV in his hand. Noninvasive monitors are placed, and general anesthesia is induced with etomidate, fentanyl, and vecuronium. After the endotracheal tube (ETT) is placed in the trachea, anesthesia is maintained with 50% nitrous oxide in oxygen with isoflurane 0.8%. Bilateral air entry is confirmed, the end-tidal CO_2 is 32 mmHg, and the end-tidal CO_2 trace looks normal. The ETT is secured. The room is darkened, as is routine in these cases. The operator (radiologist) is in close proximity to the patient's head, where he is placing an IV line in the internal jugular vein so that he can place the shunt in the portal venous system. With the x-ray machine on the other side of the head, you have no access to the airway and are unable to feel for pulses in the head or arms (the latter being tucked along side of the patient). Thirty minutes into the case, there is a sudden marked increase in the peak inspiratory pressure from 28 to 42 cm H_2O. All other parameters are within normal limits. You suspect right endobronchial intubation, but you are prevented from listening to the right side of the chest because it is made sterile and covered by sterile drapes. You are reluctant to pull the ETT back because you really do not know if there is right endobronchial intubation. Is there anything you can do to confirm your suspicions without making the surgical field on the right side of the chest unsterile?

Solution

Ask the radiologist to show you the neck and chest on the x-ray screen monitor. That is easy for him to do. If you are right, then you will see that the ETT has passed the carina into the right main bronchus. When you pull the ETT back into the trachea, you should see that the peak inspiratory pressure returns to basal levels. Furthermore, you will see that during insufflation of the lungs, the liver does not increase to the same extent with two lungs ventilation as with only right lung ventilation (1).

Discussion

During TIPS, endotracheal intubation is essential because access to the patient is severely limited. The room is dark; it is important to make sure that you have enough light in your workstation to see the monitors. This is one case in which monitors are essential, as close clinical observation of your patient is impossible. It has been recommended (1) that during such procedures, regular observation of the monitor can be beneficial to patient care. Indeed, it may be useful to tell the radiologist that he or she should also be aware of this unusual sign of one-lung ventilation.

The radiologist usually selects these patients very carefully for his procedure. Many of these patients are critically ill with sepsis and disseminated intravascular coagulation. You must always give prophylaxis for sepsis. Packed red blood cells and fresh frozen plasma should be readily available, as serious bleeding can occur from lacerations of hepatic arteries, etc. There is a procedure mortality rate in TIPS of up to 3% (2).

Recommendation

Don't forget to use the x-ray when you are worried about right endobronchial intubation during a TIPS procedure.

References

1. Eastwood N. An unusual sign of right endobronchial intubation. Anaesthesia 1995;50:90.
2. Freedman AM, Sanyel AJ, Tisnado J, et al. Complications of transjugular intrahepatic portosystemic shunts: a comprehensive review. Radiographics 1993;13:1185–1210.

25
A Tracheostomy Is Urgently Needed, but You Have Never Done One

You are called stat to the Cath lab for a patient who has developed sudden difficulty in breathing. You find a 73-yr-old woman with her neck and face severely swollen. She is unresponsive, with shallow, rapid, and labored breathing. She is receiving nasal oxygen at 4 liters/min, and the oxygen saturation is 86%. She has a diagnosis of a superior mediastinal syndrome. In an attempt to investigate this, the radiology staff sedated the patient with fentanyl 100 mg IV and midazolam 4 mg IV. With the patient adequately sedated, a Shiley catheter has been placed in the right subclavian vein. They inform you that the subclavian artery has also been hit several times, and there is now a large hematoma compressing her trachea. You listen to the chest, but can hear little air entry. You assist ventilation with 100% oxygen via an Ambu bag, to no avail. You attempt to intubate the trachea with a Mac 3 blade, but see nothing. You feel that succinylcholine will not be helpful, as the patient is now relaxed and completely unresponsive. A two-person mask ventilation with a large oral airway is unsuccessful. The laryngeal mask airway (LMA) that you called for has not arrived. The neck is so swollen that you dismiss the use of a cricothyrotomy. A tracheotomy set is produced and an ear, nose, and throat specialist is called for, but you are informed that he can only be there in 10 min. The oxygen saturation is now 76%, and there is a dramatic decrease in her pulse rate and blood pressure. Everyone is looking to you as the senior anesthesiologist. You know that you have never done a tracheotomy before under these circumstances, but feel that this is the only option for this woman. You grab the scalpel and feel a great sense of insecurity and dread, but you have committed yourself. How will you quickly secure a surgical airway?

Solution

This case happened to a colleague and I. With the thumb and middle finger of the left hand, I attempted to displace the sternomastoid muscles on either side. However, in this case, they were impossible to feel. The main reason for placing your thumb and middle finger in this manner is to protect the great vessels. With the scalpel in my right hand I made a 5-cm incision in the midline from the cricoid cartilage (which, in this case, I could not feel). The incision should traverse skin and subcutaneous tissue only. My colleague started blunt dissection of the neck with his fingers. With his fingers he opened a tract so I could barely see the trachea. With my scalpel, I cut through one of the membranes and inserted a cuffed endotracheal tube #5. With the airway secured, her oxygen saturation improved to 100% and her heart rate and blood pressure normalized. Only when satisfactory airway control was achieved did we address the bleeding, which, incidentally, was profuse. She must have lost approximately 200 ml of blood. To stop the bleeding, we packed the wound with a 2-in vaginal pack and applied pressure. The ear, nose, and throat surgeon appeared and congratulated us on a job well done. The patient survived the incident and went home after a short hospital stay.

Discussion

Moments of sheer terror do occur in anesthesia. When one is unable to ventilate and unable to intubate, one is left with very few options besides a surgical airway. The American Society of Anesthesiologists has guidelines for the management of the difficult airway (1). Although useful as an educational tool, it is just that. The introduction into the United States of the LMA in 1992 has proven to be a major advance in difficult airway management (2). However, I do not think the LMA would have helped in this case because of the swelling above and below the glottis.

Dissection of the neck by hand was the reason for this woman's survival. I initially tried to get access to the trachea with a forceps and other tools, but had to give up because of too much blood and swelling. The whole-finger dissection with insertion of the endotracheal tube took less than 1 min.

I personally don't like the cricothyrotomy or percutaneous dilatational tracheotomy. Mediastinal emphysema is a serious complication of these techniques, as they are blind (3,4). Furthermore, it is impossible to estimate the tracheal diameter.

Recommendation

A patient who has an upper airway obstruction that cannot be relieved by positive-pressure mask ventilation or bypassed by tracheal intubation or LMA placement, must have an immediate surgical airway. This could be a cricothyrotomy or a tracheotomy. The take-home message is to get access to and control the airway as rapidly as possible. Forget about the bleeding initially. The latter can be controlled by packing and pressure while you await an ear, nose, and throat surgeon. Finger dissection can save a life.

References

1. Practice guidelines for management of the difficult airway. Anesthesiology 1993;78:597–602.
2. Benumot J. Laryngeal mask airway and the ASA difficult airway algorithm. Anesthesiology 1996;84:686–699.
3. Hutchinson R, Mitchell RD. Life threatening complications from percutaneous dilatational tracheotomy. Intensive Care Med 1991;19:118–120.
4. Van Hearn LWE. Welten RJTJ, Brink RPG. A complication of percutaneous dilatational tracheotomy: mediastinal emphysema. Anaesthesia 1996;51:605.

26
General Anesthesia for a Patient with a Difficult Airway and a Full Stomach

A 26-yr-old female (American Society of Anesthesiologists physical status 2E), weight 124 kg, height 5'6", is scheduled for an emergency appendectomy. She has a class 3 airway, but tells you that she has a previous history of a traumatic and difficult endotracheal intubation. She is otherwise healthy and takes no medication. She refuses a regional block, as she has back problems. You decide on a fiberoptic intubation, but you are fully aware that topical anesthesia and sedation must be kept to a minimum in an attempt to maintain the protective laryngeal reflexes and decrease the likelihood of gastric aspiration. What approach would you adopt for this case, based on anatomical and physiological observations?

Solution

The patient should be placed in a fully upright sitting position, but with hip flexion minimized.

Discussion

Anesthesiologists often place their patients in the supine position out of habit. For this patient, there is good reason to break this habit.

Intragastric pressures in normal fasting adults may seldom reach above 30 cm H_2O (1,2). In most adults, the distance between the lower esophageal sphincter (LES) and the upper esophageal sphincter is more than 25 cm H_2O. Thus, even if the LES provides limited resistance to efflux of gastric content, it is highly unlikely that the normal intragastric pressure responsible for passive regurgitation would be sufficient to propel the gastric contents into the oropharynx in a patient sitting fully upright or even standing. The sitting position is more natural for the patient, and allows face-to-face communication with the anesthesiologist. This makes for a more relaxed patient with less need for sedation, and thus a more truly "awake" intubation.

Besides having the patient sitting up, appropriate antacid (3) and drug pretreatment to decrease gastric volume and acidity, while increasing LES tone, are considered standard of care (4–6).

Cricoid pressure is known to make fiberoptic intubation more difficult (7). There are other reasons why I would not recommend the use of cricoid pressure in these cases (8).

Adequate anesthesia of the airway should be achieved with a combination of topical and regional techniques. If regional techniques are used (personally, I don't use them), such as blocking the superior laryngeal nerves, then one must wait at least 8–10 min before instrumentation is done.

My personal recommendation for topical anesthesia in these situations is 8 ml of lidocaine 4% with 4 ml of cocaine 4%. I usually use only 6–8 ml of this solution, administered with an atomizer (Mucosal Atomizer Device; Wolfe Tory Medical, Salt Lake City, UT) or the Micromist Nebublizer (Hudson RCI, Temecula, CA), asking the patient to pant like a dog. No matter what I use, I take my time and find that I can manage with very little sedation. For sedation, I use meperidine up to 1–1.5 mg/kg, as it does not depress the ventilation like fentanyl. Also, meperidine has an atropine-like effect (9). Glycopyrrolate is also a good drug to use. I use 2 liters of oxygen flowing continuously through the suction port in the fiberoptic scope. This pushes away secretions, giving a clearer view, and provides improved oxygenation.

Recommendation

Although there are no clinical trials to support the contention that these patients should be in a full sitting position, the aforementioned theoretical considerations and years of experience indicate that this technique maximizes patient safety. In addition, it provides minimum stress and discomfort to the both patient and anesthesiologist (10).

References

1. Dow TGB, Brock-Utne JG, Rubin J, Welman S, Dimopoulos GE, Moshal MG. The effect of atropine on the lower esophageal sphincter in late pregnancy. Obstet Gynecol 1978;51:426–430.
2. Brock-Utne JG, Dow TGB, Welman S, Dimopoulos GE, Moshal MG. The effects of metoclopramide on the lower esophageal sphincter in late pregnancy. Anaesth Intens Care 1978;6:26–29.
3. Crawford S. Principles and Practice of Obstetric Anaesthesia. 3rd ed. Oxford: Blackwell Scientific Publications; 1999.
4. Andrews AD, Brock-Utne JG, Downing JW. Protection against pulmonary acid aspiration with ranitidine. Anaesthesia 1982;37:22–25.

5. Brock-Utne JG, Downing JW, Humphrey D. Effects of ranitidine given before atropine sulphate on lower esophageal sphincter tone. Anaesth Intens Care 1984;12:140–142.
6. Murphy DF, Nally B, Gardiner J. Effect of metoclopramide on gastric emptying before elective and emergency Caesarean section. BJA 1984;56:1113–1116.
7. Hunter AR, Moir DD. Confidential enquiry into maternal deaths. BJA 1983;55:367–369.
8. Brock-Utne JG. Is cricoid pressure necessary? Paediatr Anaesth 2002;12:1–4.
9. Hardman JG, Limbird LE. Goodman and Gilman's: The Pharmacological Basis of Therapeutics. 10th ed. New York: McGraw Hill; 2001.
10. Brock-Utne JG, Jaffe RA. Tracheal intubation with the patient in a sitting position. BJA 1991;67:225–226.

27
Jehovah's Witness and a Potentially Bloody Operation

A 54-yr-old (American Society of Anesthesiologists physical status 1), 79 kg, 5'11" man is scheduled for a prostatectomy. While in the operating room (OR), you hear from the circulating nurse that the patient is a Jehovah's Witness. The scrub nurse mentions that she has had a patient like this die under a similar operation. In the hope that he may take albumin, you get two bottles of 4% albumin from the pharmacy and place it on your anesthetic table behind the anesthesia machine. You meet him for the first time in the preoperative holding area. He is surrounded by 15 of his family and friends. They inform you of the patient's unbending refusal to accept blood transfusions and all related blood products. You inform the patient that you will abide by his wishes, but tell him, in no uncertain terms that he may die from hypovolemia. His response is to say he'd rather die then get blood products. You write down that you have explained the serious consequences of his refusal and get him to sign that he does not want any blood products and that he is prepared to die. You get this witnessed by as many of his family and friends that want to sign. You make a copy of this statement for your own record and place the original in the patient's chart.

His past medical history is noncontributory. He has had no previous surgeries. On examination nothing abnormal is detected and he has a class 1 airway. He is not interested in an epidural and prefers to be asleep. You place an IV, give him midazolam 2 mg IV, and take him back to the OR. The same scrub nurse and circulator nurse that you met that morning is in the OR. However, you now see that there are two circulating nurses. You introduce yourself to the new nurse whom you have not seen before. She tells you her name and says pleased to meet you. Because she is new in the OR, you presume that she is being in-serviced as a circulating nurse. The patient is placed on the OR table and you proceed to put on the noninvasive monitors. You record the baseline vital signs and start to preoxygenate the patient. The new nurse seems out of place and keeps looking at your anesthesia table behind you. You think she may be looking intently at the albumin bottles. The other circulating nurse holds your endotracheal tube and is positioned to assist you with the endotracheal intubation by the patient's head. The new nurse seems disinterested in observing what the circulating nurse is doing. You feel there is something wrong here. As you are concerned, you stop your preoxygenation and turn to the new nurse. What is it that bothers you and what would you say to her?

Solution

This situation happened to me. I stopped the preoxygenation, turned to the nurse, and asked her, "Is the patient a friend and/or relation of yours?" She blushed and muttered "No." I then said to her, "Kindly tell me if you are or are not a Jehovah's Witness?" She admitted she was and that the patient was someone she knew from the Kingdom Hall. On further questioning, she said that she had been asked by the family to observe in the OR and to make sure the patient did not get any blood or blood products. She normally worked in the hospital, but in the outpatient clinic. This was her day off. I asked her to leave; otherwise, I would have to call security to have her removed. I told her that I would not anesthetize the patient unless she left. She excused herself and left.

Discussion

There are three "take home messages" from this case:

1. It is imperative that you always know who is in the OR with you and what their reason for being there is. In this case, the circulating nurse had presumed that the nurse was new and needed to see how things were done. The circulating nurse should have made sure she knew who the other nurse was and what she was doing there.

2. Some hospitals have special forms for people who refuse blood and blood transfusion to sign. The two forms are called Conditional Refusal or Absolute Refusal (examples are shown in the next section). It is important to note that parents and/or guardians are usually prohibited by courts from making this decision for children, minors, or incompetent patients, if such refusal will threaten the life or health of the child, minor, or incompetent patient. If this situation applies, the advice of a lawyer or court may have to be obtained. Also be aware that different countries have different rules.

3. One may think that one can refuse to do the case as an anesthesiologist. Certainly that is one's right, but if you don't do it then one of your colleagues will have to do it. Will he or she thank you? I have always done these cases as they come along. However, I have managed often, when I got the patient alone, to convince him or her that conditional refusal is the way to go. If that does not work, I try to convince them of cell saver blood and/or albumin and, in most cases, they accept these options. But you can be unlucky. A very good friend and colleague lost a patient like this on the

table from blood exsanguinations. But as he said, "I was assigned this case, I did not like it, but what should I do? Give it to you?"

Recommendation

Always identify new faces that are working with you in the OR. If they don't introduce themselves and tell you what they are doing, you should introduce yourself and find out what their reason for being there is.

Below is a suggested form to be used with patients who are Jehovah's Witness:

Refusal to permit blood or blood products transfusion

I request that no blood or blood products to administered to:
_____ (name of patient).

1. Conditional Refusal.

I request that no blood or blood products be administered unless in the opinion of my physicians, serious injury or death may occur if such transfusion is not administered.

Date_____ Time_____
Signature _____
Relationship_____(Patient, parent, conservator, or guardian)
Witness_____
Witness_____

2. Absolute Refusal

I refuse to have any blood or blood products administered under any circumstances, including the possibility that death may occur if blood or blood products are not administered. This refusal is absolute.

I hereby release the hospital, its personnel, and my physicians from any responsibility whatsoever for unfavorable reactions or any untoward results due to my refusal to permit the use of blood or blood products. The possible risks and consequences of such refusal on my part have been fully explained to me by my physicians and I fully understand that such risks and consequences may occur because of my absolute refusal to receive blood or blood products.

Date_____ Time _____
Signature_____
Relationship_____ (Patient, parent, conservator, or guardian)
Witness_____
Witness_____.

28
Intraoperative Insufflation of the Stomach

During laparoscopic surgery, the surgeon often requests insufflation of the stomach. This is to check the sutures. The anesthesiologist usually does this with a large syringe attached to the proximal end of the patient's nasogastric tube. This technique has limitations, as it is difficult to maintain a certain pressure in the stomach.

The surgeon you are working with today is very demanding, as he really wants to see if the suture line is OK. He recently had two patients whose gastric sutures slipped. You bravely attempt the insufflation with your large syringe, but you fail miserably. He turns to you and says, "I don't really want to close up before I can be assured that there is no leak in my suture line. Is there nothing else you can do?"

What will you suggest?

Solution

Use the emergency jet ventilator.

Discussion

Most modern operating rooms have an emergency jet ventilator attached to the back of the anesthesia machine or directly into the oxygen wall outlet. We have used this technique for many years and found it efficient and safe (1). A 14-gauge catheter is attached to the distal end of the jet ventilator. The catheter is then placed in the proximal large lumen of the nasogastric tube. The stomach is gently distended by pressing on the lever of the jet ventilator. One can then observe the stomach being distended on the television monitor. It is important to remember that the pressure that the jet ventilator can generate is 50 psi. I always insist that the anesthesiologist practices on a surgical glove initially to get a feel for the pressure that is produced, before using it to distend the patient's stomach. There is always a theoretical potential to cause overdistension of the stomach. However, if you watch the stomach's response to your insufflation on the television monitor, this technique is both safe and efficient.

Recommendation

A jet ventilator can safely and efficiently achieve intraoperative insufflation of the stomach, to the surgeon's satisfaction.

Reference

1. Brock-Utne JG, Vierra M. Intraoperative insufflation of the stomach: another approach using a jet ventilator. Anesthesiology 1887;87:1265.

29
Sudden Intraoperative Hypotension

A 55 kg, 18-yr-old male with a history of spina bifida and developmental delay is admitted for surgical treatment of a recurrent right ischial and peroneal pressure sore. He has undergone multiple previous general anesthetics for urological problems without incident. Of special note is the fact that he has no allergy of any kind, especially no latex allergy. He is seen in the preoperative holding area, and an IV is inserted in his arm without much difficulty. The patient is very interested in the tourniquet. He is given it and he immediately starts chewing on it for comfort. He carries on chewing for approximately 30 min until anesthesia is induced. After he falls asleep it is removed. A routine general anesthetic is given, and then he is turned prone. Muscle relaxation is achieved with vecuronium 6 mg. You listen to his lungs and confirm that there is bilateral air entry. He is given Kefzol 1 g, and the operation starts. One hour after the induction of general anesthesia, the patient suddenly develops high peak inspiratory pressures (45 cm H_2O), hypoxemia (85%), hypotension (systolic 70 mmHg down from 120 mmHg), and a dramatic decrease in end-tidal CO_2. You increase the FIO2 to 1. You listen to the lungs and discover that there are no breath sounds over the left lung and only very minimal sounds from the right. The endotracheal tube (ETT) is withdrawn from 23 to 20 cm at the lips, with no change in the above respiratory findings. You now request that the patient is turned supine. When that is done, you palpate the cuff in the trachea. Peak inspiratory pressures remain elevated (over 50 cm). You can no longer feel the superficial temporal artery, indicating that you have a systolic blood pressure below 60 mmHg. The heart rate is increasing to 150 beats/min. You give epinephrine 50 mg. There is some improvement in his cardiovascular status, and the chest exam now reveals profound wheezing bilaterally. An additional 20 mg of IV epinephrine, 100 mg of IV hydrocortisone, and 10 puffs of Albuterol through the ETT causes near resolution of his bronchospasm. The vital signs return to normal. You are delighted with this turn of events, but wonder what the cause could have been for this sudden severe intraoperative hypotension. You discount an overdose of inhalation anesthetic, but you cannot ignore an allergic reaction to muscle relaxants and/or antibiotics.

Are there any other causes you would consider? If so, what will you do?

Solution

Consider a latex allergy. The suggested management of a potential latex allergy when it occurs intraoperatively is as follows:

1. Remove any latex materials. Surgeon must change gloves.
2. Ventilate with 100% oxygen.
3. Consider aborting the procedure.
4. Administer fluids.
5. Administer epinephrine 50–100 mg/kg IV bolus for hypotension and/or severe bronchospasm.
6. Take several samples of blood for Tryptase measurements (1), immunoglobulin E antibodies, and complement C3 and C4.

In our case, with the vital signs returning to normal, the surgery continued with full latex-free precautions. The operation was concluded uneventfully. Tests later revealed that the patient was highly sensitive to latex.

Discussion

Latex is the milky sap that is extracted from trees in the Amazon and used to manufacture natural rubber products. Latex products include surgical gloves, catheters, etc. So-called hypoallergenic gloves have latex in them, but in a smaller amount.

The timing of latex anaphylaxis presentation during anesthesia is from 30 to 60 min (2). This coincides with a delayed airborne exposure or with mucus membrane exposure at the beginning of the surgical procedure. In this case, which is similar to one that we have previously described (3), we believe that the extremely high exposure over a 30 min period, from chewing on a latex tourniquet, contributed to the development of the acute life-threatening latex allergy. Slater et al. (4) found that 34% of children with spina bifida had antibodies in their serum specific for latex rubber protein.

In all cases where there is a sudden cardiovascular collapse from an allergic cause, an attempt should be made to see if there is any generalized rash or flushing of the skin. Although not specific to latex allergy, it will indicate that you are dealing with a serious intraoperative anaphylaxis. Although cutaneous manifestations of latex are more common in nonsurgical cases (5), these can easily be explained by the fact that the anesthetized patients are mostly draped (6).

Lieberman (6) compared 1,158 cases of latex anaphylaxis that were not associated with anesthesia with 583 cases during anesthesia. There were no reported cases of cardiovascular collapse in nonsurgical patients, whereas surgical patients had over 50% incidence of cardiovascular collapse. Respiratory problems, on the other hand, seem more equally distributed between the anesthetized and nonanesthetized patients.

Recommendation

In this case, which is similar to a previously described case (1), we learned three things:

1. Patients with no history of latex allergy can develop a life-threatening latex allergy at any time. This is especially true in repeat urological procedures, as these patients have a high propensity to latex allergy.
2. Patients who have a potential theoretical risk of developing latex allergy should be advised and prevented from being exposed to latex products before general anesthesia.
3. Finally, all hospitals should now have all latex-free anesthetic equipment, including latex-free tourniquets.

References

1. Blanco I, Cardenas E, Aquilera L, Camino E, Arizaga A, Telletxea S. Serum tryptase measurement in diagnosis of intraoperative anaphylaxis caused by hydatid cyst. Anaesth Intensive Care 1996;24:489–491.
2. Brock-Utne JG. Clinical manifestations of latex anaphylaxis during anesthesia differ from those not anesthesia/surgery related. Anesth Analg 2003;97:1219–1229.
3. Eckinger P, Ratner E, Brock-Utne JG. Latex allergy: Oh, what a surprise. Another reason why all anesthesia equipment should be latex free. Anesth Analg 2004; 99:629.
4. Slater JE, Mostello LA, Shaer C. Rubber-specific IgE in children with spina bifida. Urology 1991;146:578–579.
5. Hepner D, Castells MC. Latex allergy: an update. Anesth Analg 2003;96:1219–1229.
6. Lieberman P. Anaphylactic reactions during surgical and medical procedures. J Allergy Clin Immunol 2001;110;S64–S69.

30
Overestimation of Blood Pressure from an Arterial Pressure Line

A 54-yr-old male (American Society of Anesthesiologists physical status 3) is scheduled to undergo an Automatic Internal Cardiac Defibrillator change under general anesthesia. His history is remarkable for coronary artery disease, hypertension, and insulin-dependent diabetes mellitus. He is 104 kg and 5'5". You meet him in the catheterization laboratory. As usual, the place is in partial darkness. You place noninvasive monitors. A right radial arterial line is secured before induction of anesthesia (Transpac IV monitoring kit; 84" disposable transducers with a 3-ml squeeze flush; Abbott Critical Care System; Abbott Laboratory, North Chicago, IL). A seemingly normal arterial waveform is present with a blood pressure of 149/116 mmHg and a mean of 129 mmHg. A simultaneous noninvasive blood pressure of 105/70 with a mean of 82 mmHg is obtained in the left arm. You change the noninvasive cuff to the right arm and get the same reading as in the left arm. The transducer is located in the midaxillary line and has been zeroed by you just before the arterial line was placed. Because you have just zeroed the transducer, you dismiss that as a cause for this difference in blood pressure reading. Furthermore, you did not see any off-set when the stopcock was opened to atmosphere.

Besides re-zeroing, what else would you do?

Solution

On closer inspection of the transducer assembly, it is noted that the stopcock lever arm is directed upward from the horizontal by approximately 15 degrees. When the lever is placed in the correct horizontal position, the arterial waveform shifted downward on the display monitor from right to left (Figure 30.1). The arterial pressure is now 100/65 with a mean of 77 mmHg, and it is similar to the values obtained from the noninvasive blood pressure measurement. The reason for this increase is that the pressure from the flush bag admixes with the arterial line pressure when the stopcock lever arm is misaligned, creating an overestimation of arterial

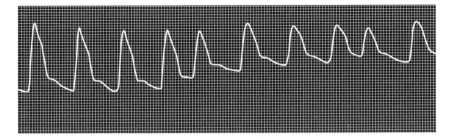

FIGURE 30.1. Right radial arterial pressure monitoring catheter showing normal appearing arterial waveform but on the right side of the trace the blood pressure is much higher (blood pressure of 149/116 mmHg and a mean of 129 mmHg). (Reproduced with permission from Eggen and Brock-Utne, 2005.)

pressure. The admixed arterial waveforms crease an artifactual waveform that appears realistic, but, numerically, is elevated. This case is akin to one previously described (1). In the darkened room, somebody may have inadvertently bumped into the transducer stopcock.

Discussion

Never work in the dark. There should be very few reasons that necessitate a darkened room when you anesthetize your patient. During the operation, it is a different matter. Based on this case, we did a study with institutional approval for human research and with informed consent. Each patient had an identical arterial monitoring set-up as in the previously described case report. Baseline waveform and pressure values were strip chart recorded. The stopcock lever arm attached to the transducer assembly was turned 90 degrees upward from the horizontal position. The stopcock lever arm was then slowly turned towards the horizontal position. At approximately 15 degrees above horizontal, an arterial-like waveform was still present, which produced a significantly higher pressure than the baseline value. When the stopcock lever arm was turned back to the horizontal, the waveform and pressure values returned to baseline (Fig. 30.1). The results of this study showed that in 8 out of 10 patients, the arterial blood pressures were artifactually increased by manipulation of the stopcock lever arm. It was noted that the degree of overestimation was in direct relation to the flush bag pressure. It was also noted that the pulse pressure of the artifactual waveform was narrower than the baseline waveform (1).

Another problem with the arterial line can be "damping," i.e., the magnitude of the difference between the input pressure and the transfused pressure. We had a case some time ago when a radial artery trace was working very well, until it suddenly plummeted to zero. The cause of our dilemma was a clamp that the nurse had used to secure wires from a microscope alongside the patient. Unfortunately, the clamp had inadvertently clamped our radial artery line (2).

Recommendation

There are many reasons for obtaining artifactual arterial blood pressure measurements. One reason is if you leave the transducer stopcock at approximately 15 degrees from the horizontal. Inappropriate treatment may be given if unrecognized. Remember that working in the dark can potentially interfere with patient care.

References

1. Eggen M, Brock-Utne JG. Artificial increase in the arterial pressure waveform: remember the stopcock. Anesth Analg 2005;101:298–299.
2. Truelsen KS, Brock-Utne JG. "Damping" of an arterial line: An unlikely cause. Anesth Analg 1998;87:979–980.

31
Severe Decrease in Lung Compliance During a Code Blue

An 80-yr-old, 90 kg, 5′7″ male with a past medical history of coronary artery disease, diabetes mellitus, right inguinal hernia, hypertension, chronic obstructive pulmonary disease, and end-stage renal disease requiring hemodialysis is admitted to an intermediate ICU with upper gastrointestinal bleeding. He is conscious, pale, cold, and clammy. Because he complains of being cold, he is covered with several blankets. His BP is 90/40 and his heart rate is 120 sinus. His hematocrit is 20 and he is transfused with 3 units of packed red blood cells over a 40-min period. After this, he becomes unresponsive, with very weak respiratory efforts. A one-stick radial arterial blood gas shows pH 6.9, pCO2 107, and paO2 53 on a 100% O_2 nonrebreather mask.

At this point, you are called to manage the airway. When you arrive, a nurse is vigorously ventilating the patient with an Ambu bag via a facemask; despite this, his O_2 saturation remains in the mid 70s. He is supine in his bed, and he is still covered with several blankets from his nipples down to his toes, with the exception of the right inguinal region, which reveals a balloon like mass. You notice this because the intern has just placed an arterial line in his femoral artery. His femoral arterial line shows a blood pressure of 80/40 mmHg and a heart rate of 120 sinus rhythm. You confirm the blood pressure is not below 60 mmHg, as you can palpate the superficial temporal artery. You turn your attention to his airway and note there is hematemesis on his pillow. You immediately place an endotracheal tube (ETT) in his trachea without sedation or relaxation. You ventilate his lungs with an FIO2 of 100%. End-tidal CO_2 is seen (Easy Cap ll CO2 detector; Nellcor, Pleasanton, CA) and bilateral breath sounds are heard. You are very concerned as you notice that the pressure required to hand-ventilate the patient is extraordinarily high and seems to get higher and higher. Unfortunately, the oxygenation only improves to the mid 80s. You repeat the laryngoscopy and confirm the correct placement of the ETT. A suction catheter is passed throughout the entire length of the ETT and no secretion of note is obtained. You give the patient vecuronium 60 mg and spray down the ETT with albuterol; there is only marginal improvement. You obtain a capnometer and confirm that CO_2 is present in the expired air and, as expected, the CO_2 trace shows an obstructive pattern. A chest x-ray has been called for, but has not been done yet. Is there anything else you would like to do, and what is the cause of the dilemma?

Solution

You undrape the abdomen. You see a very distended abdomen and the balloon-like mass in the right inguinal region points to a diagnosis of a tension pneumoperitoneum. A postintubation chest x-ray (taken after the abdomen is undraped) reveals a massive amount of free air under the diaphragm. You insert an 18-gauge angiocath into the midline, 2 cm subxiphoid. A large amount of gas is heard evacuating through the catheter. Immediately, the patient's chest compliance improves and his O_2 saturation rises quickly to 100%. His vital signs also improve, with BP 160/90 and heart rate of 90 beats/min. In a previous case report (1), the patient was extubated the following day. Investigations found no extravasation of contrast and a conservative approach was decided upon. He was discharged 15 d after his admission.

Discussion

It is postulated that the patient initially developed respiratory failure secondary to fluid overload. The vigorous mask ventilation sent much of the air into the stomach, distending it and causing an air leak through his gastric ulcer into the intraperitoneal space and into his right inguinal hernia. Despite exposure to the chest for auscultation, the abdominal distension was not obvious until the abdomen was uncovered. The abdomen should always be seen in these cases, especially in cases of perforated viscus, to alert the anesthesiologist to inadvertent pneumoperitoneum. This distention, if it had remained undiagnosed, could have proven fatal.

The blankets that covered his abdomen delayed the diagnosis of pneumoperitoneum. The main causes of accidental pneumoperitoneum are intestinal perforations (2,3). The balloon-like hernia was a clue that was missed by the medical team. However, when the blankets were removed, correct and definite treatment was instituted.

Patient draping can potentially cause a disaster in other situations, too. This can happen when, unknown to the anesthesiologist, the endoscopist injects large amounts of air into the esophagus and stomach of an anesthetized patient for better visualization. Previous reports have shown that excess air into the stomach can markedly decrease chest compliance, especially in children (4), but has also been know to do so in adults (5).

Recommendation

Always listen to the epigastric region after endotracheal intubation. If this had been done, most likely the distended stomach with the tension pneumoperitoneum, would have been discovered earlier. Also be aware of this diagnosis should you find an increased ventilatory pressure after successfully placing your ETT in the trachea when dealing with a case such as the one above.

References

1. Ternlund S, Brock-Utne JG. Failure to recognize tension pneumoperitoneum during resuscitation. Anaesth Intens Care 2006;34:517–518.
2. Ralson C, Clutton-Brock TH, Hutton P. Tension pneumoperitoneum. Intensive Care Med 1989;15:523–533.
3. Hartoko TJ, Demey HE, Rogiers PE, Decoster HL, Naglere JM, Bossaert LL. Pneumoperitoneum – a rare complication of barotraumas. Acta Anaesthes Scand 1991;35:235–237.
4. Brock-Utne JG, Moynihan RJ. Patient draping contributing to a near disaster. (desaturation during endoscopy in a 2 year old). Paediatric Anaesth 1992;2:333–334.
5. Narendranathan M, Kalam A. Respiratory distress during endoscopy- a report of an unusual case. Postgrad Med J 1987;6:805–806.

32
Shortening Postanesthesia Recovery Time After an Epidural: Is It Possible?

You are assigned to anesthetize a patient for a knee arthroscopy that is scheduled for 30 minutes. The patient is a 38-yr-old man, weight 75 kg, height 6'0", American Society of Anesthesiologists physical status 1. He is to go home the same day. He is terrified of having a general anesthetic and would like a regional block. The surgeon feels that a lidocaine infiltration of the knee joint will not give sufficient analgesia and suggests a spinal or an epidural block. Because your experience with a sciatic/femoral block is limited, you do not discuss this option with the patient. The patient is agreeable to an epidural or spinal, but states that he needs to be out of the hospital by 10 am. He is the first case of the day and you are seeing him at 7 am. You tell him that he may be in the recovery room for 2–3 h before being discharged from the hospital, as the recovery room staff has to follow standard criteria for discharge. You give him an epidural, which works fine. The surgery, commences at 7:35 am. Unfortunately, the surgery takes longer than anticipated, and the time of arrival in the recovery room is 8:30 am. On arrival in the recovery room, the patient is awake, cooperative, and with 66% motor block according to Bromage scales (1). (The scales state that inability to move toes, knees or hips equals 100% motor block; ability to move toes, but not knees equals 66% motor block; ability to partially move knees equals 33% motor block; and ability to fully move knees equals no motor block.).

You realize that you may have a problem in getting him discharged from the recovery room by 10 am. Is there anything that you can do to shorten the time he spends in the recovery room, other than having used a short-acting drug like chloroprocaine or telling the nurse that the patient can go even though he may not meet the hospital criteria for discharge?

Solution

We previously published a study where we were able to shorten the recovery time for knee arthroscopy patients by injecting 20 ml of saline into the epidural space at the end of surgery (2). No complications were noted in our study, especially due to the possibility of cephalad spread of the drug.

Discussion

Same-day discharge from the recovery room after a regional block depends on the recovery from the block. Johnson et al. (3) were the first to show that unwanted motor block caused by epidural anesthesia can be reversed by the epidural injection of saline. Unlike Johnson, who used three separate injections of 15 ml of saline, we used one 20-ml saline bolus. In our study, we found that the saline injection at the end of the surgery reduced the overall recovery room stay by 40 min. It is possible that, had we used the dosage regime suggested by Johnson et al., we may have had a different or even better result.

The mechanisms of action of this reversal are thought to be several. Neural block can be reversed in vitro by washing nerves with crystalloid solutions (4,5). Injection of epidural saline may reduce the intensity of neural block by diluting the local anesthetics (2). Local anesthetic can also be spread by the saline both caudad and cephalad. This enhances the clearance of the drug by vascular and lymphatic uptake. Removal of the drug could potentially occur because the saline 0.9% is acidic (pH 5.0). This pH change could promote ion trapping of the charged local anesthetic molecule in the epidural space.

The economic pressures are increasingly important in the delivery of surgical services. Anything that can decrease the time in the recovery room leads to decreased staffing needs. In our study (2), we speculated that this technique could save the hospital $12,650 per year if there were 10 arthroscopic procedures under epidural per week.

Recommendation

The saline epidural injection technique at the end of a surgical procedure decreases the overall length of stay in the recovery room and may have a positive impact on staffing levels.

References

1. Bromage PR. An evaluation of bupivacaine in epidural analgesia for obstetrics. Can Anesth Soc J 1069;16:46–56.
2. Brock-Utne JG, Macario A, Dillingham MF, Fanton GS. Postoperative epidural injection of saline can shorten postanesthesia care unit time for knee arthroscopy patients. Regional Anesth Pain Med 1998;23:247–251.

3. Johnson M, Burger G, Mushlin P, Arthur GR, Datta S. Reversal of bupivacaine epidural anesthesia by intermittent injections of crystalloid solutions. Anesth Analg 1990;70:395–399.
4. Gissen A, Covino B, Gregus J. Differential sensitivities of mammalian nerve fibers to local anesthetic agents. Anesthesiology 1980;53:467–474.
5. Benson H, Gissen A, Strichartz G, Avram AJ, Cavino BG. The effect of polyethylene glycol on mammalian nerve impulses. Anesth Analg 1987;66:553–559.

33
Difficult Airway in an Underequipped Setting

You find yourself in a foreign land on a medical mission with plastic surgeons repairing facial deformities. As the only anesthesiologist, you are in charge of the anesthesia equipment. You are requested to anesthetize a large man (180 kg) for removal of scars from his face. His neck circumference is over 40 cm. You would like to do a fiberoptic intubation, but the patient is terrified and wants to be asleep. You realize that you may need to have a gum elastic bougie as a backup, but discover, to your dismay, that there are none available. You start looking for possible ways of making a bougie from what you have available. The 18-French nasogastric tube would be too soft and the suction catheters you have are too short. Is there anything you can do to make the nasogastric tube stiffer and thereby use it as a bougie?

Solution

The nasogastric tube, with some modification, can be used as an alternative to the gum elastic bougie (1). The modification consists of placing one part of a paper clip into the distal orifice of the nasogastric tube via the small air vent channel and advancing proximally. The distal end of the paper clip is then pushed into the distal blind pouch of the air vent channel to minimize any danger of inadvertent trauma by the paper clip. The other end of the nasogastric tube is then cut, leaving the remaining tube with the clip 60 cm long. The end of the nasogastric tube, with the clip in it, is bent to a desired curvature and the whole tube is placed in a basin full of ice. Within a minute, the now converted nasogastric tube is rigid and can be used as a bougie.

Discussion

This solution is meant to assist anesthesiologists only in a third-world environment when they find themselves without a bougie and need to manage a potentially difficult airway. Only by working in the third world can one begin to understand the enormous difficulties and frustrations that our colleagues in these places face on a daily basis (2).

An 18-French nasogastric tube is suitable for 8-mm and larger endotracheal tubes (ETTs), whereas the 14-French tube can be used for 6–7-mm ETTs. Nasogastric tubes have the added advantage over a gum elastic bougie because they can be converted into jet stylets, thereby providing oxygen. This can be done by inserting a 14-gauge intravenous catheter (Cathlon IV; Criticon, Tampa, FL) into the proximal end and attaching it to a transtracheal jet ventilation system. For the 18-French nasogastric tube, the catheter should be inserted all the way to the neck to ensure an adequate seal. The nasogastric tube can also be used to provide oxygen to the spontaneously breathing patient with the help of a standard 3-mm ETT adaptor for the 18-French size and a 2.5-mm ETT adapter for the 14-French size. When the adapter is inserted into the proximal end, the tube can be attached to a conventional anesthetic circuit to insufflate oxygen.

Recommendation

This alternative to a bougie may prove useful when a difficult endotracheal intubation is anticipated and no other adjuncts to secure the airway are available. The added advantage of the nasogastric tube is that it allows one to insufflate oxygen.

Please review Chapter 12 for history and how to successfully use the bougie.

References

1. Manos SJ, Jaffe RA, Brock-Utne JG. An alternative to the gum elastic bougie and/or the jet stylet. Anesth Analg 1994;79:1017.
2. Manos SJ, Jaffe RA, Brock-Utne JG. Airways, paper clips and nasogastric tubes. Anesth Analg 1995;81:208–209.

34
Delayed Cutaneous Fluid Leak After Removal of an Epidural Catheter

You are called after hours to evaluate clear liquid leaking from an "epidural catheter puncture hole." The patient is a 50-yr-old Asian male (American Society of Anesthesiologists physical status 2) who had an exploratory laparotomy with gastrostomy for gastric cancer 5d before. He had an epidural catheter, through which epidural hydromorphone had been used until the 2nd postoperative day, when it was removed intact. The patient is sitting up in bed and not complaining of anything, not even a headache. His past history and examination are noncontributory.

On examination, the dressing applied to the area of the leak is soaked, and the patient's bedding is very wet. At the site of an L4–5 puncture, clear liquid is dripping out of the puncture site at a rate of about 10–12 drops/min. Closer inspection of the patient's back reveals evidence of minimal dependent edema. How would you proceed to establish whether this is cerebrospinal fluid (CSF) or subcutaneous edema fluid without resorting to computed tomography scan, radionuclide myelography, or measurements of CSF specific isoenzymes?

Solution

You collect fluid from the puncture hole and send it for analysis of glucose, chloride, and protein. At the same time, you insert an 18-gauge intravenous catheter 4cm lateral to the epidural site and insert it 1cm into the tissues. In a previous study (1), fluid was seen dripping from that site too. Fluid was again collected and the values obtained were found to be similar to the ones obtained from the lumber puncture site. A diagnosis of subcutaneous edema fluid leak was made from the puncture hole. The computed tomography was canceled, and the CSF-specific isoenzymes were not done (2).

TABLE 34.1. Comparison of various biochemical values for differentiating CSF and interstitial fluid.

	Glucose mmol/liter	Chloride mmol/liter	Protein g/liter	Ach
Plasma	4.4–6.6	90–110	60–80	–
CSF	2.75–4.12	122–132	0.15–0.45	CSF-specific enzyme
Interstitial fluid	3.85–6.05	95–105	60–80	Nonspecific enzyme

Discussion

Table 34.1 shows a comparison of various biochemical values for differentiating CSF and interstitial fluid.

CSF fluid/cutaneous fistulae are known to occur after trauma, surgery, and infections. On the other hand, fistulae secondary to subarachnoid of epidural punctures are very rare (3,4). In our case, the correct diagnosis was made without resorting to expensive tests. It is important to realize that all CSF fistulae previously reported had occurred within 48h after the removal of the catheter. We were very anxious about this case, as a CSF leak of this magnitude through a small cutaneous fistula would have required a substantial increase in CSF pressure. Others have recommended a lumbar puncture to obtain a CSF sample in similar cases (5). This is not recommended, as increased intracranial pressure may be present. A diagnosis of a CSF cutaneous fistula may require special radioisotope myelography (6) when sufficient fluid cannot be obtained. If the suspected fluid can be collected in adequate quantity (0.5ml), simple chemical analysis can avoid time-consuming, and often expensive, diagnostic tests (1,5). If the chloride and glucose values for the fluid are ambiguous, then the collected fluid can be tested for CSF-specific acetyl cholinesterase (2). This may occur when CSF mixes with interstitial fluid as it travels through the fistula.

Recommendation

This simple, inexpensive, and rapid test can prove whether the problem is caused by CSF or interstitial fluid. Expensive and time-consuming tests may prove to be totally unnecessary.

References

1. Ennis M, Brock-Utne JG. Delayed cutaneous fluid leak from the puncture hole after removal of an epidural catheter. Anaesthesia 1993;48:317–318.
2. Vanner RG. Acetylcholinesterase – a specific marker for cerebrospinal fluid. Anaesthesia 1988;43:299–300.

3. Jawalekar SR, Marx GF. Cutaneous cerebrospinal fluid leakage following attempted extradural block. Anesthesiology 1981;54:348–349.
4. Morparia HK, Vontivillu J. Case report: Cerebrospinal fluid fistula – a rare complication of myelography. Clin Radiol 1991;44:205.
5. Downey L, Slater EM, Zeitlin GL. Differentiating interstitial fluid from cerebrospinal fluid. Anesthesiology 1985;63:120.
6. Liberman LM, Tourtellotte WW, Newkirk TA. Prolonged post-lumbar puncture cerebrospinal fluid leakage from lumbar subarachnoid space demonstrated by radio isotope myelography. Neurology 1971;21:925–929.

35
Traumatic Hemothorax and Same-Side Central Venous Access

A 35-yr-old woman is admitted to the emergency room after attempting suicide by jumping from a bridge. She is in severe pain, but orientated for time and place. Her heart rate is 120 beats/min and her BP 85/40. She is breathing 100% oxygen through a nonrebreathing mask with safety vent. (Hudson RCI, Temecula, CA) and her oxygen saturation is 96%. She has multiple fractures, including pelvis, right humerus, 9th thoracic vertebra, and ribs 6–10 on the right side. She has a right-sided hemothorax. The right subclavian vein is cannulated using the infraclavicular approach and the Seldinger technique. A cordis catheter (PSI kit; Arrow International, Inc., Reading, PA) is inserted and blood is easily withdrawn for chemical analysis, internal normalized ratio (INR), and cross matching for 6 units of red blood cells. After inserting the right chest drain, 1,500 ml of blood is drained rapidly without any ill effects. A new chest x-ray shows complete resolution of the hemothorax and the subclavian catheter is seen in the correct place. The central venous pressure (CVP) is zero and fluctuates with respiration. Blood arrives, and 4 units of packed red cells are given rapidly through the subclavian vein via a Level 1 Fluidsystem warmer 1000 (Level 1 Technologies, Rockland, MA). The emergency room staff is concerned because despite continuous volume replacement with 3 liters of crystalloids and albumin 250 ml × 4 through a 16-gauge IV catheter in her right hand, her blood pressure deteriorates and increased drainage of dark blood is seen from the chest drain. A diagnosis of laceration of major vessels in the chest is made, and you are called to anesthetize this patient for a right thoracotomy. You place two additional cannulae into the right internal jugular and right femoral veins. Blood is easy withdrawn from both catheters. You attach the subclavian vein to a CVP monitor, which again shows a value of zero and fluctuates with respiration. More blood is given through the new large-bore catheters and the patient seems to stabilize. Dark blood is still draining out of the right chest drain but at a slower rate. The laboratory reports that the international normalized ratio (INR) is 2.3. The surgeon orders fresh frozen plasma. You are still looking at the dark blood coming out of the chest drain and wondering about the increased INR, as clinically she does not seem to be oozing. You send off a repeat INR. The surgeon is keen to start the operation and you agree reluctantly, but you feel there is something wrong. Why are you concerned?

Solution

This case is similar to one reported earlier (1). At thoracotomy, minimal bleeding is found, but the subclavian catheter is lying in the pleural cavity. As blood had been given only through the subclavian vein catheter, the color of the drained blood did not raise any suspicion, although it was noted to be very dark. However, the increased INR (the sample taken from the subclavian vein) indicated that the initial blood sample had come from the hemothorax. The repeat INR from the femoral vein showed a normal value of 1.1.

Discussion

Central venous catheter is useful for assessing fluid balance and for rapidly administering large volumes of blood and fluid. Blood reflux and respiratory fluctuations are considered reliable signs of correct placement of the catheter. However, this has been questioned (1–3). This would especially be true if the central venous catheter is inserted on the same side as the hemothorax and/or blood has already been transfused through the catheter. In these cases, reflux of blood and/or respiratory fluctuation of venous pressure with respiration, may not always be reliable signs to confirm correct placement of the central catheter.

It is suggested that, in these cases, blood is taken for INR estimation immediately, and put into a glass tube to observe clot formation. If there is no clot within 15 min, then you should consider whether the catheter may be in the pleural space. If you are concerned, you should observed the chest drain, in particular looking for a correlation between changes in the rate of drainage and the rate at which the fluid is infused through the catheter. The composition of both should be compared for similarities in dilution, volume, and/or color, particularly if substances like methylene blue are being transfused. If possible, the central line on the same side as the hemothorax should not be used for blood transfusion. This avoids confusion and possible wastage of blood (2). Injection of methylene blue into the central line will make the diagnosis of a pleural catheter easier.

Despite the above problem, I recommend that you place the central lines on the same side as the hemothorax. However, you need to be aware that such problems as described in the above case may arise.

Recommendation

When a central venous line is placed inadvertently in the pleural space, reflux of blood, fluctuation with respiration, and even radiological control, can be misleading. A quick way to confirm a catheter in the pleural space is to take a sample of the patient's blood from the CVP catheter into a glass tube to observe clot formation. If the clot does not form within 15 min, then the catheter may be in the pleural space

References

1. Daschmann B, Sold M, Bodendorfer G. Blood reflux, central venous cannulation and right sided hemothorax. Anaesthesia 1992;47:629–630.
2. Pina J, Morujao N, Castro-Tavares J. Internal jugular catheterization. Blood is not a reliable sign in patients with thoracic trauma. Anaesthesia 1992;47:30–31.
3. Parse MH, Tabora F, Al-Sawwaf M. Monitoring: vascular access techniques. In: Shoemaker WC, ed. Textbook of Critical Care. Philadelphia: W.B. Saunders; 1989:139–141.

36
Single Abdominal Knife Wound?
Easy Case?

A 23-yr-old man (75 kg and 6′0″) is admitted with a single stab wound just below his umbilicus. There are no other injuries as per the emergency physician. The patient is conscious, orientated for time and place, and vital signs are stable. He states he has not eaten anything for 6 h, but he smells of alcohol. Blood is taken for hematocrit and chemical analysis, and it is cross-matched for blood. His history is noncontributory. He has no allergies, and a previous general anesthetic for a right inguinal hernia repair is reportedly uneventful. The surgeon wants to do an emergency laparotomy and the patient is taken to the operating room at 9 pm, where you meet him for the first time. You review the chart and confirm his history. On examination, the patient has one stab wound, as described, and no other injuries as far as you can see. A 16-gauge IV in his left hand is working well. Examination of the anterior part of his chest and heart reveal nothing abnormal. You elect to do a rapid sequence technique, using thiopental and succinylcholine. Before induction, the blood results become available and his electrolytes, creatinine, and blood glucose are all within normal limits. His hematocrit is 36%. Normal routine monitors are placed, including a three-lead electro-cardiogram, a noninvasive blood pressure monitor on his right arm, and an oximeter on his left ring finger. You give the patient 1 g of Keflex slowly (over 2–3 min) IV, as ordered by the surgeon. The test dose of Keflex is negative, as there is no change in hemodynamic parameters. You note the vital signs and start to preoxygenate the patient. General anesthesia is induced with thiopental 200 mg, succinylcholine 100 mg, and an endotracheal tube (ETT) is placed uneventfully in the trachea. You hear bilateral air entry and end-tidal CO_2 is present. The ETT is taped at 22 cm and the surgery begins. Anesthesia is maintained with fentanyl 250 mg and isoflurane 0.8%, with 50% oxygen in air. Shortly after the incision is made, there is a rapid decrease in this systolic blood pressure to 40 mmHg. His heart rate goes to 150 beats/min and the saturation falls to below 82%. You ask the surgeon to check for bleeding, but he states that there is no bleeding in the abdomen. He also feels the diaphragm and states that it is intact. By now, the end-tidal CO_2 is nearly at zero, despite the fact that you can hear bilateral air entry over the anterior part of his chest. You tell the surgeon to do a thoracotomy, but the surgeon feels this must be an allergic reaction or an anesthetic mishap. Large doses of epinephrine are given IV, with no improvement. Despite heroic attempts on your part and those of your colleagues who come to help, the patient is pronounced dead 30 min later. If the patient did not die from an allergic response to drugs, from an anesthetic mishap, or from an undiagnosed surgical bleed in the abdomen, why did the he die?

Solution

This happened to a friend of mine. At postmortem, a stab wound that had been missed was found in the left axilla. The pericardial sack was full of blood and there was a large ragged wound in his left ventricle and left atrium.

Discussion

The most important thing to realize is that if a patient with one stab wound is alive, then there is another stab wound. Usually, a patient with one stab wound is dead only if the murderer is an assassin or an expert in killing people with a knife. In my experience, I have never seen only one stab wound in a patient who is alive.

Patients with stab wounds, or bullet wounds for that matter, must all be examined properly before anesthesia. Sitting the patient up and examining every part of the patient is imperative, otherwise bad things can happen.

Recommendation

A patient with one stab wound that is alive has one or more wounds somewhere else. You must examine your patient thoroughly in these cases, otherwise death can occur.

37
A Draw-Over Vaporizer with a Nonrebreathing Circuit

You are the only anesthesiologist who is part of a medical team to visit an outlying village in Columbia, South America. Unfortunately, all your anesthetic equipment has not arrived and today is the day for operations on 12 orthopedic patients. You are presented with an Ohmeda Cyprane PAC (portable anesthesia complete) isoflurane draw-over circuit as the only available anesthesia delivery system (Fig 37.1). The anesthesia nurse, who is a Columbian and works in the hospital, says she had been recommended this equipment by an overseas anesthesiologist some years ago. She has used it with great success both for spontaneously breathing patients and those she had to paralyze. In the latter case, she used an Ambu bag attached to the draw-over circuit. She tells you that she was recommended to use the Penlon Oxford Ventilator (which was also left behind) instead of the Ambu bag. However, she has not used it yet. She is very keen for you to show her how to use the Penlon Ventilator. You are not so sure, but ask for any information she may have on this equipment. She hands you a paper (1) describing the use of the draw-over vaporizer and the Penlon Oxford Ventilator (the latter is to be placed at F in Fig. 37.1). You read the text and study the diagram below. The vaporizer D is fitted with a 900-ml corrugated anesthetic tubing (B) with a dust filter at the inlet (A). Oxygen can be given through inlet C. Air is drawn in and through the vaporizer by the patient during inspiration. B acts as a reservoir of oxygen between inspirations if oxygen is used. However, in a healthy patient you may elect not to use oxygen. The outlet E of the PACU vaporizer incorporates a one-way valve that is connected via a second anesthetic tube to a T-connector (F). This T-connector is the ventilation port to which an Ambu bag or a ventilator can be attached. From the T-connector right exit, another anesthetic tube leads to a one-way Ruben's valve (G) and the patient's mask (H), or to an endotracheal tube. An exhaust tube (I) carries expired gases from the patient to a scavenging system or into the air. A side-stream adaptor (J) is used for end-tidal CO_2 and/or gas analyzer. Unidirectional flow during ventilation is maintained in the PAC draw-over circuit by the one-way valves at E and G, such that negative pressure at F draws only carrier gas through the vaporizer and into the circuit. Positive

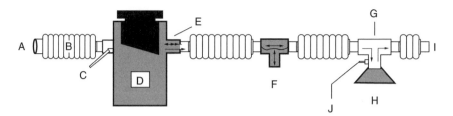

FIGURE 37.1. The Ohmeda Cyprane PAC isoflurane draw-over circuit (Ohmeda, Madison, WI). For explanation see text. Reproduced with permission from Ali and Brock-Utne JG, 1992.

pressure applied at F directs the flow only to the patient, as reverse flow is blocked at E. Back flow of exhaust gas into the circuit is also blocked during all phases of respiration by the Ruben's valve. You also discover that the Penlon Oxford Ventilator is fed by a compressed gas source, and thus provides only a positive-pressure cycle.

You have read all this, but you are still concerned that combining the PAC vaporizer and the Penlon Oxford ventilator may not work as intended. What should bother you about marrying these two items?

Solution

In a previous study (2), we showed that the Penlon ventilator did not provide any vapor to a test lung. This is explained by the fact that the Penlon Ventilator is only fed by a compressed gas source, and thus provides only a positive-pressure cycle. Therefore, it is impossible to draw any carrier gas, and therefore any vapor, from the vaporizer (Fig. 37.2).

Discussion

When this anesthetic circuit is used with a draw-over vaporizer for controlled ventilation, it is essential to use a self-inflating bag or ventilating equipment that can draw the carrier gas through the vaporizer and into the circuit to ensure delivery of the anesthetic gases. A previous study (1) mentioned that this ventilator can be used with a draw-over vaporizer circuit. It is obvious that awareness may occur if the Penlon is used as recommended (1). Because the Penlon ventilator uses compressed gas, it is not useful in a situation where no compressed gas is available. Hence, under these circumstances, manual ventilation may be the only means available if the patient needs to be paralyzed.

In our study (2), we also found that attaching an Ambu bag incorrectly at position A led to the production of a vapor concentration dangerously

CIRCUIT FLOW

PENLON VENTILATOR AT POSITION "F"

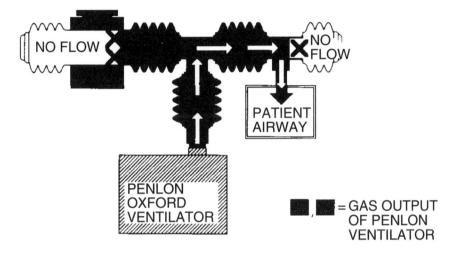

FIGURE 37.2. Penlon ventilator attached at position F. This ventilator provided only a positive-pressure cycle and was unable to draw any carrier gas (and, therefore, vapor) through the vaporizer. When this ventilator was attached at position A, ventilation produced excessive airway pressures and vapor concentrations dangerously in excess of the vaporizer settings. Ventilation port A is not recommended by the manufacturer. Reproduced with permission from Ali and Brock-Utne JG, 1992.

in excess of the vaporizer settings. In addition, the distal one-way valve (G) became stuck, creating extremely high pressures to the patient airway.

Recommendation

When faced with anesthesia delivery systems that you have never used or seen, it is imperative that you be aware of the pitfalls and problems that can occur when using this equipment.

References

1. Ezi-Ashi TI, Papworth DP, Nunn JF. Inhalational anesthesia in developing countries. Part 2. Review of existing apparatus. Anaesthesia 1983;38:736–747.
2. Ali K, Brock-Utne JG. Performance evaluation of a draw-over vaporizer with a non-rebreathing circuit during stimulated adverse conditions. J. Clin Anesth 1992;4:468–471.

38
Unexpected Intraoperative "Oozing"

A 64-yr-old woman (American Society of Anesthesiologists physical status 3) is scheduled for a craniotomy for clipping of a large aneurysm. Her history includes hypertension, obesity (130 kg and 5'6"), and insulin-dependent diabetes mellitus. She is alert and orientated and moves all limbs. She claims her exercise tolerance is good, meaning that she can walk half a flight of steps without stopping or getting breathless. The size of the aneurysm worries the surgeon. Therefore, he has requested that a femoral arterial sheath be placed by the neuroradiology team in the femoral artery before the surgical incision. The reason for this is that, should clipping of the aneurysm prove to be impossible or dangerous, coiling of the aneurysm can then be attempted via the femoral artery. You anesthetize her in a routine manner and the anesthetic proceeds according to plan with stable vital signs. The interventional radiologist cannulates the femoral artery. After that, he infuses the femoral sheath with a heparinized solution (500 ml normal saline with 2,000 units of heparin) under pressure via a pressure bag (Infusable Pressure Infusor; Vital Signs, Totowa, NJ). The solution drips very slowly into the femoral artery via a 60 drops/ml Piggyback Microdrip with a Clair clamp controlling the rate (1–2 drops every minute) (LifeShield; Hospira, Inc., Lake Forest, IL). There is no transducer system attached. The patient is turned 180 degrees from the anesthetic machine and the surgery begins. After 90 min, the aneurysm is exposed. The surgeon complains that there is a lot of oozing in the surgical site and that he has difficulty maintaining adequate hemostasis. He asks you if the preoperative coagulation was normal. You answer that it was and tell him that the liver enzymes were also within normal limits. He says, "Please give her some fresh frozen plasma (FFP) and tell me when you have given it." You are at a loss to understand the cause of the oozing, but order the FFP as soon as possible. You send off new coagulation studies (international normalized ratio, prothrombin time, and partial thromboplastin time) and an arterial blood gas (ABG). You also place 5 ml of her blood in a glass tube. The results from the ABG, including electrolytes and blood sugar, come back within normal limits. However, the blood in the glass tube is still liquid, even after 15 min.

Five minutes later, the FFP arrives and you infuse it quickly. The surgeon reports no improvement. You tell him that you are still waiting for the coagulation results from the lab. You are at a loss to understand what is going on, and the surgeon is unhappy. What do you think could be the cause of the oozing, and what will you do?

Solution

You check the bag with the heparinized solution that is being infused into the femoral artery. You discover to your dismay that the 500 ml bag is totally empty. You immediately do an activated clotting time (ACT) and discover that it is prolonged. You inform the surgeon and give protamine IV, which quickly reverses the effect of the 2,000 units of heparin that had inadvertently been infused. The clipping of the aneurysm is concluded successfully and the patient makes an uneventful recovery. This case is similar to a previously reported case (1).

Discussion

This case highlights the importance of keeping a watchful eye on all health care personnel performing procedures on anesthetized patients under your care. In this case, the interventional radiologist did not use a transducer system to keep the femoral artery patent. Instead, he relied on a simple IV line with a stopcock controlling a pressurized heparinized saline bag. When we discovered that the cause of the intraoperative oozing was due to the excess heparinized saline solution given through the femoral sheath, we closed it, and replaced their IV set with our own transducing system.

In our case report (1), we did note that no transducer system was being used, but did not think it was important. That was a big mistake. We now routinely hand the interventional radiologist our transducer system when they insert a femoral sheath.

Laboratory coagulation studies do take time and the shortcut to place some blood in a plain glass tube is a good one. You will know within 10–15 min whether you have a problem. This test is very useful during obstetric emergencies and trauma where disseminated intravascular coagulation can develop. The result from this test is usually available up to an hour before the laboratory coagulation studies are available. Hence, you can start the disseminated intravascular coagulation treatment much earlier.

Recommendation

Two points are worth noting about this case:

1. Keep a watchful eye on all health care personnel working on anesthetized patients.
2. Understand the limitations and potential problems of equipment and/or techniques that other health care providers use.

Reference

1. Chung A, Brock-Utne JG. Similar invasive procedures, but different techniques. (A potential disaster). Can Anaesth J 1999;46:999.

39
Central Venous Access and the Obese Patient

You are scheduled to anesthetize a 54-yr-old, 160 kg, 183 cm tall (body mass index = 47.8 kg/m^2) man with vasospasm for cerebral angiography. He had been admitted to the intensive care unit 3 d earlier, after an emergency craniotomy for a subarachnoid hemorrhage. When you meet him in the radiology suite, he responds sluggishly to verbal commands, but reacts to pain. His heart rate is regular at 66 beats/min, and the blood pressure is 160/90. The neurosurgeon is happy with that pressure. An endotracheal tube had been removed 12 h previously. He is breathing spontaneously on an oxygen mask, providing 2 liters of oxygen per min. His vital signs are within normal limits. His only IV access is a triple-lumen right subclavian venous catheter (16 cm long) (Arrowgard Blue Plus Multi-lumen CVC; Arrow International, Inc., Reading, PA). This had been inserted at the time of the original operation. Through the proximal lumen of this catheter, IV propofol 100 mcg/kg/min is being infused for sedation. Via the medial lumen, neosynephrine 200 mcg/kg/min is given for pressure support. Maintenance fluid is given through the distal port. You review the previous anesthesia team's note in their anesthesia record. They report no problem with airway management. Despite that, you make sure you have a fiberoptic cart, bougie, etc., available. You check the anesthetic machine and make sure your anesthesia equipment and all your anesthesia drugs are ready. You call for a colleague to come and give cricoid pressure. He arrives and you look set to start the anesthetic. However, is there something else that you should do before induction of general anesthesia?

Solution

You should always check the patency of any IV you are using before induction of a general anesthetic. This is especially true when you using someone else's IV. We recently had a case like this (1). In that case, we could aspirate blood from the distal end of the triple-lumen catheter, but not from the other ones. Because we were in the radiology suite, contrast medium was injected in all three lumens under direct fluoroscopic control. The only lumen that was noted to be intravascular was the distal lumen. Propofol (proximal lumen) and neosynephrine (medial lumen) were both seen to extravasate into the subcutaneous tissue of the neck. Rather than pulling this catheter out, we placed, under fluoroscopic control, a long guidewire into the right atrium through the distal lumen. The triple-lumen catheter was removed, and a double-lumen catheter (20 cm long), which was also made by Arrowgard, was inserted over the guidewire. After that, we used fluoroscopy with dye injection to confirm later that both lumens were in the vein. Anesthesia was induced uneventfully and the patient was taken back to the intensive care unit in stable condition.

Discussion

The triple-lumen catheter, which was originally placed to its hub, was 16 cm long. The patient had a large neck (>70 cm in circumference) and due to the distance between his skin and the vein, only the distal lumen was intraluminal. The replacement catheter was 20 cm long, and the additional length was needed to allow both lumens intravenous access. We could have used the 20-cm-long triple-lumen Arrowgard, but it was not available at the time.

Because peripheral IV access may be limited in obese patients (2), cannulation of a central vein (subclavian or internal jugular) is often recommended for IV access (3). A problem similar to the one described in this chapter has been reported with a much shorter 10.8-cm pulmonary artery catheter introducer in an obese patient (4).

Of interest was the fact that the blood pressure in the right arm was very different from the left. The systolic blood pressure in the right arm was 20 mmHg higher than in the left arm. When checked 24 h later, the blood pressure in the two arms were equal. This temporary difference is attributed to the subcutaneous infusion of neosynephrine.

Recommendation

It should always be your routine to ascertain the patency of the IV before induction of general anesthesia. This is especially true for central lines. When using any multilumen catheter, all lumens should be checked to confirm patency after initial placement. Remember that in morbidly obese patients, catheter position can change with movement (4), so intravascular position must be confirmed periodically in these patients.

References

1. Ottestad E, Schmiessing C, Brock-Utne JG, Kularni V, Parris D, Brodsky JB. A complication of central venous access in an obese patient. Anesth Analg 2006;102:293–294.
2. Juvin P, Blarei A, Bruno F, Desmonts J-M. Is peripheral line placement more difficult in obese than lean patients? Anesth Analg 2003;96:1218.
3. Johnson G, Tobias JD. Central venous access in morbidly obese patients. Anesth Analg 2001;93:1363.
4. Thompson EC, Wilkins HE III, Fox VJ, Fernandez LG. Insufficient length of pulmonary artery introducer in an obese patient. Arch Surg 2004;139:794–796.

40
Taking Over for a Colleague: Always a Potential Concern

You are just out of residency and have joined your first general practice group. This evening you are on fourth call. There is nothing for you to do, so you are told to leave. Just then an emergency laparotomy is booked. The patient is morbidly obese with an acute abdomen. She is 4 d out after a gastric bypass procedure. You offer to help and the first call accepts your offer. The patient arrives in the operating room within 5–10 min. She complains of severe abdominal pain. Her respiratory rate is over 40 and shallow. Her heart rate is 130 sinus tachycardia, with a blood pressure of 100/60. She has a cold periphery, and her oxygen saturation is 91% on room air. The patient is placed on the operating table with a ramp, as previously described (1), to improve your view on laryngoscopy. Preoxygenation and a rapid sequence induction commence. You provide cricoid pressure. The anesthesia-induction drugs are given by your colleague. It appears to you that your colleague is using fentanyl, etomidate, and rocuronium, in that order, for anesthetic induction. You see no fasciculation. Your colleague performs the laryngoscopy and tells you that he has a grade 1 view. The endotracheal tube is seen to pass between the cords and bilateral air-entry is heard. An obstructive end-tidal CO_2 pattern is seen. For general anesthesia maintenance, isoflurane is added to the oxygen. At this point, your colleague is called urgently to another room where there is a code blue. You say you will stay and look after this case. He leaves in a hurry. You place the patient on the ventilator and the vital signs, including the respiratory parameters, are stable. However, the heart rate is still 130 sinus tachycardia. You start getting ready to place an internal jugular vein line, but the oxygen saturation is seen to fall to 88% from 98%. The airway pressure has risen from 40 to 56 cm H_2O. You start to ventilate the patient manually and notice that it is very difficult to do so. It has now been 5–6 min since the anesthetic induction. The airway pressures continue to be high, but the saturation is improving. You listen to the chest and confirm bilateral equal air-entry. You pass a suction catheter down the whole length of the endotracheal tube without any problem. Sucking on the catheter yields no secretion. Because the oxygen saturation is improving, you place the patient back on the ventilator. Unfortunately, the peak pressures are still high (58 cm H_2O) and the oxygenation saturation starts to fall again. The patient is not moving and the pupils are pinpoint. You are at a loss as to what to do next. You can feel the pressure mounting in the room, as everyone is looking at you and wondering what the "new boy" is going to do. What will you do?

Solution

You look at the syringes that are still stuck in the line attached to three-way stopcocks. To your surprise you see the syringe that you thought was rocuronium is actually labeled succinylcholine. You draw up some rocuronium and give 80 mg. Within 2 min, the ventilator airway pressures falls and the oxygenation improves.

Discussion

When assisting a colleague with a case, it is imperative to know what he or she is doing and what drugs are being administered. Remember that when you are taking over a case after it has begun, you must make sure that your anesthesia machine is working. Because you have not had the opportunity to check it before the case, if your colleague has not done so, you could get into trouble. I have seen several near misses with this scenario.

Recommendation

When you don't know what is going on, always check your facts. In this case, information as to what drugs had been given proved vital for safe patient care. If you had known it was succinylcholine, then you would have given a nondepolarizing muscle relaxant and this problem would never have occurred.

Reference

1. Collins JS, Lemmens HJM, Brodsky JB, Brock-Utne JG, Levitan RM. Laryngoscopy and the Morbid Obesity: a comparison of the "sniff" and "ramped" positions. Obesity Surg 2004;14:1171–1175.

41
Intraoperative Epidural Catheter Malfunction

A 62-yr-old obese male (120 kg, 190 cm tall, body mass index 33.2 kg/m²), American Society of Anesthesiologists physical status II, is scheduled for a colectomy secondary to ulcerative colitis. You plan a combined general anesthetic technique with an epidural. When the patient is in the operating room, you place an epidural catheter (20-gauge closed tip) (B. Braun Medical, Inc., Bethlehem, PA) uneventfully in the L4-5 interspace. The length of the epidural catheter in the epidural space is 4 cm. As is your practice, the epidural catheter, as it leaves the patient's back, is led in a semicircle over a folded 2 × 2 inch swab. This is then covered with an OpSite (Flexigrid; Smith and Nephew, Hull, England). The catheter is attached to the patient's back and over his right shoulder using Compound Benzoin Tincture U.S.P. (The Clinipad Corporation, Guilford, CT) and tape (Hytape Surgical Produce Corporation, Yonkers, NY). There is a negative test to 3 ml of lidocaine 2% with epinephrine 1:200,000. A total of 22 ml of lidocaine 2% is then injected and a block to T-4 is achieved. The patient is placed in a supine position and routine general anesthesia commenced. Two additional boluses are injected into the epidural space with good effect and no problem. Forty minutes after the last dose, the surgeon requests that the patient be placed in a steep head-down position. Shortly thereafter, it becomes impossible to inject anything through the epidural catheter, despite the use of a small syringe. You suggest that the surgeon puts the table back in the original position, but he is unwilling to do so at that time. You are reluctant to abandon your epidural. Is there anything else you could do to get the epidural to function adequately again?

Solution

We have previously described two such cases in obese patients (1). The solution we discovered was the following. One of us placed both hands underneath the patient's lumbar and thoracic area and pulled the catheter, tape, and the subcutaneous tissue towards the head. The other person, at the same time, attempted to inject lidocaine into the epidural space with a syringe. Immediately after the catheter/tape was pulled cephalad, the plunger descended into the syringe. This indicated that the catheter was functioning again. The patient remained pain-free for the next 18 h. At 18 h the catheter had stopped working. We attempted again to do the traction maneuver, but this was unsuccessful. The epidural catheter was removed. On examination of the nonfunctioning epidural catheter, we discovered that a 4-mm section of the catheter was severely narrowed. The narrow section was 22 cm from the tip. Attempts to inject saline through this catheter, after its removal from the epidural space, were unsuccessful. It is possible that our last attempted forceful traction, applied to tape and tubing, caused this severe narrowing of the catheter. Hence, the traction maneuver should not be done with excessive force.

Discussion

This is another example of an anesthetic complication that can occur in obese patients that are under your care. An intraoperative epidural malfunction is a real problem for patient care because a change in an anesthetic plan must be made if the epidural can't be made functional again. We speculated that, in our case, the steep head-down position caused the catheter to be kinked or stretched so that it temporary occluded the lumen. A total obstruction of an epidural catheter has been reported in the postoperative period (2). In that case (2), the catheter became severely stretched and permanently obstructed when the patient was moved from the operating room table to the trolley. It was made functional again by cutting the catheter distal to the stretched portion and reattaching the catheter connection. The stretching of an epidural catheter leading to an obstruction has also been reported on the withdrawing the Tuohy needle over the catheter (3). To prevent this from occurring, the needle should be withdrawn slowly and in line with the catheter. An epidural catheter can also become kinked at the point of entry into the supraspinous ligament, if the insertion of epidural is done with the patient in a very flexed position. When the patient then straightens out, the catheter gets obstructed (4). An epidural catheter can also be knotted in the epidural space (5). This probably occurs when the catheter forms a loop in the epidural space, then doubles back on itself and forms a knot. These authors recommend that the catheter should not be introduced more than 2.5 cm into epidural space. However, the majority of anesthesiologists leave the epidural catheter at least 3 cm in the space (6).

Manual stretching (pulling the catheter with both hands) of a Braun epidural catheter shows that an enormous force must be produced before damage to the catheter is seen (1).

Recommendation

It may be prudent, in obese patients, to initially tape the epidural catheter laterally to the midaxillary line, and thereafter in front of the arm to the shoulder region. In this way, the movement of the subcutaneous tissue of the back is less likely to kink, stretch, or bend the catheter. In the recovery room, the catheter can be retaped.

References

1. Leith P, Sanborn R, Brock-Utne JG. Intraoperative epidural catheter malfunction in two obese patients. Acta Anaesthesiol Scand 1997;41:651–653.
2. Smith AJ, Eggers KA. Potential hazard with the epidural space catheterization. Anaesthesia 1995;50:88–89.
3. Khalour FK, Kunkel Fa, Freeman J. Stretching with obstruction of an epidural catheter. Anesth Analg 1987;66:1202–1203.
4. Wildsmith JAW, Armitage EN. Principles and Practice of Regional Anesthesia. 2nd ed. New York: Churchill Livingstone; 1993.
5. Nash TG, Openshaw DJ. Unusual complication of epidural anaesthesia. Br Med J 1968;1:700.
6. Gough JD, Johnston KR, Harmer M. Kinking of epidural catheters. Anaesthesia 1986;4:1060.

42
Breathing Difficulties After an Electroconvulsive Therapy

You are scheduled to do an outpatient electroconvulsive therapy (ECT) on a 36-yr-old female. This is her fourth ECT in a series of at least eight. She tells you that the previous ones have been uneventful and that her mood is better. She is 90 kg, and 5′6″ in height. She works in her husband's restaurant, where she is a cook. Her medical history is significant for depression, hypertension, insulin-dependent diabetes mellitus, and hypothyroidism. She takes nifedipine, enalapril, insulin, thyroxine, paroxetine, and fluphenazine. After she arrives in the treatment room, an IV is started. You examine the patient and find nothing abnormal, including her airway exam. Her chest is clear to auscultation. Her heart rate is 90, BP 130/70, respiratory rate is 12, and room air oxygen saturation is 97%. You place noninvasive monitors on the patient and start to preoxygenate her. Anesthesia is induced with etomidate 16 mg, followed by succinylcholine 1 mg/kg. The patient is hyperventilated and the ECT procedure is done uneventfully, except excess salivation is noted after the treatment. The patient awakens from the anesthetic, but suddenly sits up and starts to cough violently. Her saturation falls to 86%. You diagnose laryngospasm and provide positive-pressure mask ventilation with 100% oxygen. After a few minutes, the laryngospasm is broken and she is now breathing easier. She sits up, and although her oxygen saturation is now 96% on nasal oxygen (6 liters/min,) she complains that she does not get enough air. (The nurse tells you now that this difficulty with breathing happened last time she had an ECT, but she slowly improved and was discharged home.) The nurse tells the patient to lie down, but she refuses. She again states that she can't breathe. She rips off all her monitors and refuses to have them replaced. The nurse tells you she did that last time too. Are you concerned, and if so what will you do?

Solution

If you are worried, then stay worried. In this case, with all the monitors off, you correctly examine the patient's chest and cardiovascular system. This case is similar to one we have previously described (1). In that case, we found that the patient had bilateral crepitation over both lung fields. A chest x-ray showed moderate pulmonary edema and a diagnosis of negative-pressure pulmonary edema (NPPE) was made. The patient was given furosemide 20 mg. One hour later, there was a rapid clinical improvement. She was admitted for observation and discharged home the next day. The patient found the complication frightening and elected not to return for further ECTs.

Discussion

Oswalt et al. (2) were the first to describe this complication. The pathophysiology of NPPE has been outlined, but the exact mechanism has not yet been defined (3). Two conditions must be present for NPPE to be produced: inspiratory air obstruction, and strong spontaneous inspiratory efforts. Is it noteworthy that NPPE can develop in a matter of seconds. The main differential diagnosis is pulmonary aspiration mimicking the signs of NPPE (i.e., hypoxia and decreased compliance). However, the presence of these signs after correction of airway obstruction in a spontaneously breathing patient merits the presumptive diagnosis of NPPE. If frothy, pink fluid appears, the diagnosis is almost certainly correct. In our patient, the clinical examination, the chest x-ray, and the rapid resolution of her symptoms with treatment, helped confirm the diagnosis.

In our case (1), we postulated that excess secretion, most likely caused by a large dose of succinylcholine, resulted in laryngospasm, followed by pulmonary edema. There is really no need to give more than 0.5–0.7 mg/kg of the drug to prevent the breaking of bones during the ECT. The routine use of glycopyrrolate or atropine might have prevented this complication. However, anticholinergic medications may exacerbate the tachycardia associated with ECT. But bear in mind that when I started anesthesia, atropine was routinely given prior to ECT because of the concern of bradycardia/ cardiac standstill. This is, of course, present in a proportion of ECT patients.

At this time, there is no way of clinically predicting who will develop NPPE. However, it is more likely to occur in strong healthy adults (4).

Recommendation

If you are worried about your patient, stay worried, even though you are told this happened before and there seems to be nothing to worry about. You should always examine your patient and make your own assessment. This is, after all, your patient. Although NPPE is uncommon, being aware of this complication allows for early recognition and prompt treatment.

References

1. Cochran M, DeBattista C, Schmiesing C, Brock-Utne JG. Negative-pressure pulmonary edema: a potential hazard in patients undergoing ECT. J ECT 1999;15:168–170.
2. Oswalt CE, Gates GA, Holmstrom F. Pulmonary edema as a complication of acute airway obstruction. JAMA 1977;238:1833–1835.
3. Loyd JE, Nolip KB, Parker RE, Rosellie RJ, Brigham KL. Effects of inspiratory resistance loading on lung fluid balance in awake sleep. J Applied Physiol 1986;60:198–203.
4. Goitz RJ, Goitz HT, DiFazio CA, McCue FC, III. Identification of acute pulmonary edema following routine outpatient orthopedic procedures in healthy, young adults. Orthopedics 1994;17:949–952.

43
White "Clumps" in the Blood Sample from an Arterial Line: Are You Concerned?

You are scheduled to anesthetize a 67-yr-old woman for a lower abdominal resection of a rectal cancer. She has a history of coronary artery disease, hypertension, obesity, and insulin-dependent diabetes mellitus. A previous anesthetic 6 mo before for a laparoscopic cholecystectomy was, according to the patient, uneventful. You have no previous anesthetic record to refer to. She proves to be a difficult IV stick, but you manage to put a 20-gauge IV in her hand. You sedate her and take her to the operating room. Prior to induction of anesthesia, you place an arterial line in the patient's right radial artery. This is connected to a pressure transducer containing 1,000 U heparin in 500 ml of normal saline. Thereafter, you position the patient sitting up and place an epidural for postoperative pain relief. The test dose is negative and, again, the patient is placed supine. Anesthesia is induced uneventfully with etomidate, sufentanil, vecuronium, and isoflurane in air. Because the patient has very poor IV access, you elect to put in a central line. A right internal jugular catheter is placed uneventfully and is seen to work well. The surgery starts and you elect to send an arterial blood sample to the laboratory for estimation of the usual parameters, including blood sugar. To your dismay you note that white "clumps" precipitate out of the sample. You repeat the test and find the same result. However, blood from the central line does not show any "clumps." You are wondering if you should be worried about this and if so why?

Solution

This is an example of heparin-induced thrombocytopenia (HIT), also known as heparin-induced thrombocytopenia-thrombosis syndrome (HITTS) (1,2). Heparin is now recognized as the leading cause of drug-induced thrombocytopenia in the perioperative period (2). Platelet aggregation or clumping is the primary mechanism, leading to the development of life-threatening thrombotic events in cerebral and myocardial circulation. It is also known as the "white clot syndrome" (2).

In the case mentioned above, the outcome was disastrous. The HIT panel came back positive. The platelet count dropped from 153,000 to 23,000 and the patient suffered a stroke on the first day postoperatively, from which she never recovered. This was thought to be due to the severe cerebral thrombosis, as spontaneous intracranial bleeding is considered rare. We attempted to publish this case in 2002, but were told by various editors that there was nothing new in our submission. At that time, I would contend, that HIT and its serious complications were not well known.

Discussion

It is important to remember that the HIT reaction can occur in patients who have previously received heparin without any problems, just like latex allergy (3). Patients with a previous diagnosis of HIT/HITTS should have no heparin or heparin analogs under any circumstance. These include heparin-coated catheters, lovenox, or other low-molecular weight heparins, heparin flushes of catheters, and subcutaneous heparin. The following drugs should be used as alternatives if anticoagulation is required:

1. Bivalirudin (Angiomax). This is given 0.15–0.20 mg/kg/h without an initial bolus. It is broken down enzymatically and excreted via the kidney. Its half-life is 25 min.
2. Argatroban (Novastan outside of USA). The dose is 2 mcg/kg/min, without an initial bolus. The drug is excreted via the liver and has a half-life of 40–50 min. It is interesting to note that the drug increases the INR, so one must aim for a higher therapeutic range.
3. Danaparoid sodium (Orgaran). This drug is currently unavailable in the US because there have been rare cases of crossover reactivity with anti-heparin antibodies.
4. Lepirudin (Refludan). Recombinant hirudin. The drug is given as a bolus 0.4 mg/kg, and the infusion is 0.15 mg/kg/h. The drug is excreted by the kidney and the half-life is 80 min, with normal kidney function. In kidney failure, the half-life rises considerably.

So, should heparin be removed as a drug to prolong vascular patency? In a study by Tuncali et al. (4), they found that no statistically significant difference in pressure waveform dampening and arterial occlusion after catheter decannulation. However, they did identify the risk of vascular occlusion. This could be correlated with the presence of a hematoma at the puncture site, the duration of cannulation and the age of the patient. They concluded that the use of heparin flush solution did not improve the arterial catheter patency in the perioperative period. Until definitive evidence is available, the routine use of heparin flush solution in vascular access should be considered carefully in both adults and children (1).

In conclusion, proper positing of the arm, nursing care of the catheter, and continuous normal saline flush under pressure may prove to be adequate to maintain patency, especially in high-risk patients (1).

Recommendation

In a case where you suspect the patient is developing HIT, you immediately do the following:

1. Stop all heparin and heparin-containing products, including low–molecular weight heparin and heparinoids.
2. Send a blood sample to the laboratory asking for HIT tests. These are the heparin-induced platelet aggregation assay (HIPAA) and the ELISA test for heparin_PF4 antibodies. It is important to note that if the first test comes back negative you carry on treating the patient has if he/she has HIT and send another test. If that is also negative then carry on and monitor for possible delayed HIT for at least 24 h. The ELISA test can give a 15% false negative rate, but if the platelet count is dramatically down from a normal baseline the patient should be treated as if he/she has HIT.
3. If anticoagulation is required, then use alternatives to the heparin. Warfarin (Coumadin) must never be used, unless a direct thrombin inhibitor is given first to maintain anticoagulation. Warfarin alone can precipitate a massive thrombosis caused by depletion of proteins C and S (2).
4. If possible, avoid platelet transfusions. There is a higher risk for these patients to develop thrombosis than to start bleeding. This is seen even in the face of significant thrombocytopenia. Platelet transfusion can lead to significant thrombosis in these cases (3).
5. Early intervention with a heparin substitute may minimize the permanent damage from thrombosis.
6. The patient must be told that he or she has a heparin allergy. A wristband and a sign over the bed should warn everyone of this drug allergy. Lastly, this allergy must be recorded in the patient's medical record.

References

1. Chow JL, Brock-Utne JG. Minimizing the incidence of heparin-induced thrombocytopenia: To heparinize or not to heparinize vascular access? Ped Anesth 2005;15:1037–1040.
2. Warkentin TE, Greinacher A. Heparin-induced thrombocytopenia and cardiac surgery. Ann Thorac Surg 2003;76:2121–2131.
3. Eckinger P, Ratner E, Brock-Utne JG. Latex allergy: oh what a surprise. Another reason why all anesthesia equipment should be latex free. Anesth Analg 2004;99:629.
4. Tuncali BE, Kuvaki B, Tuncali B, Capar E. A comparison of the efficacy of heparinized and nonheparinized solutions for maintenance of perioperative radial artery catheter patency and subsequent occlusion. Anesth Analg 2005;100: 1117–1121.

44
Anesthesia for a Surgeon Who Has Previously Lost His Privileges

You have just completed your residency and joined an anesthesia group that has many surgical locations to cover. Today, you are assigned to a free-standing surgical clinic. This is your first time at this clinic. Your first case is a 42-yr-old male who is a drug abuser and positive for HIV. According to the surgical history and physical exam, he is otherwise healthy. He is scheduled for a cervical discectomy under monitored anesthesia care (MAC). Upon arrival at the clinic, you introduce yourself to the head nurse. She tells you that the surgeon always does these cases under MAC and has refused in the past to have them done under general anesthesia. You look at the operating room list and discover that this is (fortunately) the only case he is doing today. You arrive in the change room and one of your anesthesia colleagues tells you that the surgeon you are working with today has lost his privileges in many hospitals and clinics in the area. He also lost his privileges in the one you are in now, but has recently been reinstated. This is his first time back after a 12-mo absence. You ask why he lost his privileges in this clinic and you are told that he punctured the trachea in one patient during a cervical discectomy under MAC. This led, in the postoperative period, to severe surgical emphysema of the neck with obstruction of the airway. Even though he was aware that the patient had breathing difficulty due to surgical emphysema in the postoperative period, he did nothing and left the hospital. The patient stopped breathing 30 min later. Without the timely intervention by an anesthesiologist, the patient would have died. Adding to your concern is the fact that you are told that the surgeon told the patient to sue the anesthesiologist, as it was his fault. You are now really apprehensive and wonder what you should do. What would you do?

Solution/Discussion

There is no simple solution to this problem.
There are 3 options:

1. You should remind the surgeon that you have the right to provide an anesthetic technique that you think is the safest for this patient. You have no doubt that this case must be done under general anesthesia, with an endotracheal tube. Should the surgeon refuse your anesthetic plan then you can refuse to provide the anesthetic. If he agrees to a general anesthetic and you do it, but are concerned at the end of the case that the surgeon may have traumatized the trachea, then you could remove the endotracheal tube over a tube exchanger or bougie (1). Should your patient develop respiratory complications that necessitate rapid reintubation, you can use the tube exchanger or the bougie.

2. You can delay this case (patient has a cold, etc.) and give yourself time to confirm that the surgeon has had his privileges restored. One would hope that the administration of any hospital or clinic would check before they allow him to schedule a case. In addition, if you reside in California, you can ask for the surgeon's medical record from the California Board of Medical Quality Assurance. If he has lost his privileges for what you consider is well below the standard of care, then you can approach the administrators of the surgical clinic with your anesthesia colleagues to discuss your concerns.

3. In most academic centers, you have the right to refuse to work with a specific surgeon, just as he has the right to refuse to work with you. However if you do refuse, then one of your colleagues will be asked to do it, and I doubt that they will thank you. In private practice, the situation can be very different. In the latter case, your anesthetic group may have a contract with a hospital/surgical clinic to provide anesthesia care. Hence, you may not be in a situation to refuse to do the case, as it could be seen as a break in contract. However, if you decide to do the anesthetic, then it must be as you want it. No surgeon should dictate to you what anesthetic the patient should have, nor should we dictate to them how their surgery should be done.

Recommendation

Always do what is best for the patients, even if this means you do not follow the surgeon's preference for the type of anesthetic. In a case such as this one, if you manage to cancel the case, then you can check if the surgeon has indeed lost his privileges and if they have been reinstated. Information as to why he lost his privileges can prove to be vital to you and your anesthesia group's future association with this surgeon and/or the clinic that supports him.

Reference

1. Robles B. Hester J. Brock-Utne JG. Remember the gum-elastic bougie at extubation. J Clin Anesth 1993;5:329–331.

45
Airway Obstruction in
a Prone Patient

Today you are anesthetizing a 58-yr-old man (82 kg and 5'11") with a cerebellar tumor. He is otherwise healthy and classified as an American Society of Anesthesiologists physical status 2. General anesthesia is induced uneventfully and the patient is turned prone after having been placed in a Mayfield pin holder. The patient's head is 180 degrees away from the anesthesia machine. The neck is flexed so that there is a 1-finger gap between the mentum of the mandible and the sternal notch. You would prefer to have 2 fingers, but the surgeon says he needs the flexion to do the operation. The operation proceeds uneventfully for 6 h, when there is an increase in the peak inspired pressure from 24 to 42 cm H_2O over a 2–4 minute period. All the other parameters have not changed. You call for help, and one of your colleagues comes to your aid. With his help you confirm bilateral air entry with no adventitious sounds. You inspect the endotracheal tube at the mouth and confirm that it has not moved and is still taped at 22 cm H_2O. Your colleague places the patient on 100% oxygen and after a few minutes you attempt to pass a suction catheter through the endotracheal tube (ETT), but it only goes in 15–20 cm. You manipulate the ETT, but there is no improvement. Your colleague suggests you let the endotracheal cuff down (the cuff could have herniated into the lumen), but even then you are unable to pass the suction catheter. You diagnose a partial kink in the ETT. The vital signs are still within normal limits, but the peak airway pressure has gone down to 48 cm H_2O. You are concerned. You can now ventilate the patient, but should the kink be total this could have serious consequences for the patient. There are 30–45 min left and the surgeon is unhappy to reposition the patient's neck before the end of the surgery and about your request to turn the patient supine and reintubate the trachea. You get a laryngeal mask airway ready in case you are unable to ventilate the patient. What else could you do to improve the ventilation without extending the neck or turning the patient supine?

Solution

Replace the angle connector at the end of ETT with a Bronchoscopic Swivel Elbow adaptor (PriMedico, Largo, FL) (*see* Chapter 12 for a picture of the Bronchoscopic Swivel Elbow). Through the bronchoscopic port (at the top end of the connector) you advance a gum elastic bougie or semirigid Sheridan Jet Ventilation Catheter/tracheal tube exchanger (Rusch, Inc., Duluth, GA) (R.G. Dacanay and B.W. Mecklenburg, written communication, 2004) or a Cook's exchange catheter (Cook Critical Care, Ellettsville, IN). With these three devices you should be able to straighten the kink. With the two latter devices you can ventilate, using the orifice in the middle of the Sheridan Jet Ventilation Catheter or the Cook's exchange catheter.

Discussion

Sudden airway obstruction in a prone patient can end in disaster. The above solution can be lifesaving. This is especially true if the neck is flexed to a significant degree. Many years ago I had an episode where the ETT fell out onto the floor from the mouth of an anesthetized prone patient. Luckily, the head was in a neutral position and I managed to intubate the trachea by placing myself on the floor under the head of the patient. With the laryngoscope in the right hand, I found it very easy to place the ETT with my left hand.

Recommendation

An obstructed airway in the prone patient is fortunately rare, but the suggested solutions may prove to be lifesaving in these critical situations. To have a Bronchoscopic Swivel Elbow Adaptor available in these cases may prove to be invaluable.

46
A Question You Should Always Ask

You are just out of residency. Today you are scheduled to do a laparo-scopic tubal ligation. The patient is a 28-yr-old diabetic with an insulin pump placed. She had a baby boy 2 wk earlier and now wishes to have her tubes tied. Otherwise, she is healthy, weighs 118 kg, and is 5′6″. You meet the patient for the first time in the preoperative area and discover to your dismay that the insulin pump is on. She has been fasting since the night before. You check the blood sugar and find it is 25 mg%. By now you have a working IV and you are infusing 50 ml of 50% dextrose. An epidural for her delivery had been a great success, and she wonders if she can have the same again. You explain to her that because the surgeon will be distending her peritoneal cavity with gas and tilting her head down it will be difficult for her to breath. She will also get a "referred pain" to her shoulder, which could be very bad and which an epidural would not prevent. The surgeon does not want to do a local with some sedation, and he leaves you with two options: either a general anesthetic or an epidural/spinal.

You elect to do an epidural. The surgical procedure goes uneventfully and the patient is very grateful. How did you get away with doing an epidural in this case?

Solution

This situation happened to me when working in private practice. The surgeon, when asked how long he was going to be responded, "Less than 15 min." Actually, the operation took only 13 min from skin to skin. However, at 10 min, while in full Trendelenburg, the patient complained of severe bilateral shoulder pain. She had no pain from the abdomen. At that point she was placed supine, the abdominal incision was closed, and the shoulder pain subsided over a 2-min period.

Discussion

It is always important, especially when you don't know the surgeon, to enquire how long he or she will be. The way I recommend you deal with this matter is to say: "Where I trained, the surgeons were known to take over an hour (or whatever) to do this case." So when the surgeon responds and says he will be 15 min you not only get valuable information but also make the surgeon feel good.

Recommendation

If you don't know your surgeon, it is imperative to find out what they are going to do and how long they think they will be.

47
Postoperative Vocal Cord Paralysis

You are scheduled to anesthetize a 65-yr-old woman (American Society of Anesthesiologists physical status 2) for a left carotid endarterectomy (CEA). She has hypertension, which is well controlled medically. Her past surgical history is significant for a thyroidectomy 17 yr ago. Otherwise she is well, with no known allergies. Her physical exam is normal and she has no stridor or hoarseness. She prefers to be awake for the surgery, and you do a deep and superficial cervical plexus block with 1.5% lidocaine with 1:200,000 epinephrine. Six milliliters is injected at C3, C4, and C5, while 14 ml is injected into the superficial plexus. The surgery starts with the patient awake, as she has only received midazolam 2 mg and 50 μg of fentanyl for the block. After a Pilling retractor is inserted, pushing the internal jugular vein and sternocleidomastoid laterally and the thyroid and trachea medially, the patient coughs repeatedly. The surgeon injects 6 ml of plain lidocaine 1% around the common carotid artery, but this does not help as the patient now develops stridor and becomes agitated. The retractor is removed and within a few minutes she feels much better. The surgeon inserts the retractor again, but once again the patient develops severe coughing and stridors. The patient is told that a general anesthesia is needed and she reluctantly agrees. She is anesthetized without any problems with fentanyl 200 ug, etomidate 18 mg, and vecuronium 7 mg. She is easy to mask ventilate. You have a grade 1 view, and your resident does note that the right vocal cord seem closer to the midline than the left. You have a look and agree with his assessment. An endotracheal tube (ETT) is placed uneventfully. The anesthetic is maintained with oxygen-nitrous-isoflurane. The surgery is completed uneventfully and a special note is made by the surgeon that the vagus nerve is intact. There is no evidence of a nonrecurrent laryngeal nerve. The recurrent laryngeal nerve is not seen.

At the end of the surgery the surgeon is happy for you to just remove the ETT from the trachea. You are concerned about the vocal cord mobility and hence a bit hesitant to remove the ETT. What should your "modus operandi" be in this case?

Solution

To assess the vocal cord mobility, the patient is allowed to breath spontaneously on sevoflurane after the effect of vecuronium is reversed by glycopyrrolate and neostigmine. With the patient deeply anesthetized and breathing spontaneously on sevoflurane, the ETT is removed. The patient is breathing unaided with minimal evidence of airway obstruction. Immediately thereafter, a #3 laryngeal mask airway (LMA) is inserted and a fiberoptic bronchoscopic (FOB) is inserted through the LMA. In a case similar to this one (1), bilateral vocal cord adduction (vocal cord paralysis) with moderate supraglottic edema was seen. An ear, nose, and throat (ENT) surgeon recommended that a tracheostomy be done, especially in view of the supraglottic edema. Serial FOB performed on days 2 and 5 after the tracheostomy, revealed bilateral vocal cord paralysis. On the ninth day, movement of the left vocal cord was noted. The tracheostomy was removed 2 wk after the surgery, and the patient made an uneventful recovery.

Discussion

Airway obstruction after CEA can occur from several causes, including tissue edema, nerve injury, and neck hematoma (2).

In this case (1), the authors postulate that the right recurrent laryngeal nerve was damaged during the thyroidectomy done many years previously. This led to paralysis of the right vocal cord. As long as the left vocal cord was working, the patient had no complaints and the physicians were unaware of this problem. However, when during this surgery the left vocal cord was temporarily paralyzed, the effect was acute bilateral vocal cord adduction and acute stridor.

Thyroid surgery is reported to lead to permanent and/or transient palsy of the vocal cords in 1–2% of patients (3), whereas the incidence of unilateral vocal cord paralysis under CEA is reported to be up to 6% (4).

Recommendation

A patient who is coming for a CEA after a thyroidectomy should preferably have an ENT evaluation of the vocal cords before surgery.

References

1. Kwok AOK, Silbert BS Allen KJ, Bray PJ, Vidovich J. Bilateral vocal cord palsy during carotid endarterectomy under cervical plexus block. Anesth Analg 2006;102: 376–377.

2. O'Sullivan HC, Wells DG, Wells GR. Difficult airway management with neck swelling after carotid endarterectomy. Anaesth Intesive Care 1986;14:460–464.
3. Rosato L, Avenia N Bernante P, et al. Complications of thyroid surgery: analysis of a mulitcentric study on 14,934 patients operated on in Italy over 5 years. World J Surg 2004;28:271–276.
4. Mniglia AJ, Han DP. Cranial nerve injuries following carotid endarterectomy: an analysis of 336 procedures. Head Neck 1991;13:121–124.

48
A Serious Problem

You are a new attending anesthesiologist at a university hospital. It is late in the evening and you are on second call. A craniotomy has been ongoing for 4 h and there is 1 h to go. Your resident (32-yr-old married male), although competent, does not seem particularly interested in what you are trying to teach him. You have worked with him before, but at that time he had seemed much more interested and willing to learn. Today, he also complains about being cold, although you feel warm. He is wearing a long-sleeved gown. He has been to the rest room at least three times in this period. He now wants to go again. You ask him if there is anything wrong, and he states that he is fine, but needs to go to the bathroom. He is in the rest room when your colleague, who is first call, comes into the operating room (OR) to send you home. You tell him about the case and remark to the first call that the resident seems to have TB (tiny bladder). He tells you that this has been his impression also. No more comments are made and you leave the OR. As you get into the corridor, a nurse comes running toward you shouting that there is a person unconscious in the hallway. You run to the scene. Here you find your resident collapsed on the floor. He is cyanotic and not breathing. With a firm jaw trust he starts to breath, albeit slowly. His vital signs are within normal limits, but he still unconscious. You pinch his arm and he pulls the arm away. You are very concerned and call for more help. Aided by the nurse, you quickly establish an IV with Lactate Ringer. You give him an ampoule of 50% glucose as you think he may be hypoglycemic, but there is no improvement in his consciousness level. What will you do?

Solution

This happened to me. When help came, another colleague discovered that his pupils were pinpoint. He was taken to the emergency room where a tox-screen was positive for narcotics. The next day he was in the chairman's office and then sent onto a treatment center. After treatment was completed, he was permitted back to the department to continue his residency.

However, after another episode with drug abuse, he decided to change specialties. As far as I am aware, he is still alive.

Discussion

The definition of drug addiction, as defined by the American Society of Anesthesiologists, is:

The overwhelming compulsion to use drugs in spite of adverse consequences. It is a chronic, progressive disease that results in loss of control of one's life. Unless it is recognized and treated skillfully, addiction will result in disability and will often end with death. Physical dependence frequently develops but is not present in all drug addictions.

Although the exact rate of substance abuse among physicians is unknown, conservative estimates are that 8–12% of physicians will develop a substance abuse problem at some point during their career (1). Drug abuse has been shown to be a major risk factor for medical malpractice and negligence lawsuits (2), the development of physical and psychological illnesses, and adverse effects on the family (3). This does not take into account the harm that can be done to the patient and to the profession as a whole. It is a fact that physicians with substance abuse problems often remain undetected for many years before any intervention is made, and by then it may be too late (4). Left untreated, the mortality rate among drug abusing physicians has been reported to be as high as 17% (5). Anesthesiologists are thought to be especially at risk (6), but this has been questioned (1).

I have known five anesthesiologists who died after giving themselves a drug overdose. Three died in the hospital while on duty, and two died at home using propofol and/or thiopental. Of these five, two had been known to use anesthesia drugs to excess in the past, but despite that they were allowed to practice anesthesia. Another six (including the case above) were discovered before they killed themselves, and they were sent to treatment centers. Of these six, three were residents who managed to complete the anesthesia residency. I have lost contact with these six. I do know that one had a relapse while in private practice, but is doing fine now.

Recommendation

The American Society of Anesthesiologists has produced two very good pamphlets entitled: "Chemical Dependence Guidelines for Departments of Anesthesiology" and "Chemical Dependence In Anesthesiology." In the latter booklet is a list of what to look for to identify a potential drug-abusing physician. Among these are:

1. Charting that becomes increasingly sloppy and unreadable.
2. Preference to work alone.
3. Unusual behavior changes, i.e., mood swings, with periods of depression followed by euphoria.
4. Difficult to find between cases, as he takes short naps.
5. Requests frequent bathroom breaks.
6. Wears long-sleeved gowns to hide needle sticks.
7. Often states he is cold, and hence, wears long-sleeved gowns.
8. Pinpoint pupils.
9. Patients anesthetized by a drug abuser, may complain of pain that is out of proportion to the amount of narcotic charted on the anesthetic record.

References

1. Cicala RS. Substance abuse among physicians: What you need to know? Hosp Physician 2003;20:39–46.
2. Rivers PA, Bae S. Substance abuse and dependence in physicians: detection and treatment. Health Manpow Manage 1998;24:183–187.
3. Boisaubin EV, Levine RE. Identifying and assisting the impaired physician. Am J Med Sci 2001;322:31–36.
4. Brown RL, Flemming MF. Training the trainers: substance abuse screening and intervention. Int J Psychiatry Med 1998;28:137–146.
5. Bohigian GM, Croughan JL, Sanders K. Substance abuse and dependence in physicians; an overview of the effects of alcohol and drug abuse. Mo Med 1994;91;233–239.
6. Spiegelman WG, Saunders L, Mazze RI. Addiction and anesthesiology. Anesthesiology 1984;60:355–341.

49
A Leaking Endotracheal Tube in a Prone Patient

You are to anesthetize a 30-yr-old man (91 kg) who is donating his bone marrow to an unknown person. He is classified as an American Society of Anesthesiologists physical status 1 with a class 1 airway. The patient has had no previous anesthesia/surgery and his family history is negative for anesthesia-related complications. He takes no medication and has no drug allergy. An IV is placed in his left hand and midazolam 2 mg is given in the preoperative holding area with good effect. He is anesthetized in a routine manner and mask ventilation is uneventful. After the airway is secured with an endotracheal tube, the patient is turned prone. His head is turned to the side so that you can see both eyes. Everything is progressing as planned until 10 min before the end, when you notice that there is a progressive leak in the endotracheal tube (ETT) cuff. You are eventually unable to blow up the cuff. The patient's vital signs remain stable, but the oxygen saturation has decreased from 100% to 96%. The peak pressure has fallen from 36 to 22 cm H_2O.

You inform the surgeon and suggest that you change the ETT either with a tubechanger or by turning the patient supine. The surgeon tells you that he has only a few more minutes to go. Is there anything else you can to do to enable you to stop the leak in the cuff and thereby ventilate the patient adequately?

Solution

The problem can easily be rectified by packing the throat with a 2-in moist vaginal pack (1). This was done and the surgery was completed uneventfully.

Discussion

The use of a vaginal pack can be extremely helpful in these cases. They are especially useful in cases where the cuff develops a leak after a successful, but difficult, endotracheal intubation. Your reluctance to remove a correctly placed ETT in these circumstances is understandable. Changing the ETT over a tube changer could be dangerous. Packing the throat, and thereby sealing the leak, may prove to be the safest move when facing a similar situation.

The use of these packs to "buy time" in the emergency room can prove lifesaving. The pack can then be used to stabilize the patient's vital signs before you change a leaking ETT. I have used this technique in the emergency room many times. It occurs with regular monotony in the ER when you arrive to secure the airway. You are handed a laryngoscope and an ETT. The ETT you are given is invariably bloody and the cuff damaged by the patient's teeth from previous attempts at laryngoscopy. I always select my own ETT and check it, but there are times when you have no such luxury and a rapid endotracheal intubation is called for.

Recommendation

The throat packs come in two sizes: 1 in or 2 in. Moisten the pack in water and squeeze the water out. Tie a single knot in what is to be the distal end of the pack. This is done to tell you when the pack has been completely removed. Because it is rare that you place a throat pack, I make it a rule to always write "PACK" on a piece of tape and place it on the patient's forehead or ETT. In this way, I prevent leaving a pack behind when I remove the ETT.

Reference

1. Vickery IM, Burton GW. Throat packs for surgery. Anaesthesia 1997;32:565–572.

50
Lessons from the Field: Unusual Problems Require Unusual Solutions in Impossible Situations

You are stationed in a cottage/mission hospital in Africa as the anesthesiologist. You are called to anesthetize a 35-yr-old healthy male who has been stabbed in the neck with a wooden knife. You run to the emergency room and find the patient in stable condition. He is awake and cooperative. The wooden knife's handle is visible sticking out of his neck with the wooden blade disappearing under the clavicle, directed toward the heart. He is otherwise healthy, with no previous surgeries or allergies to drugs. The surgeon wants to remove the knife under general anesthesia. You send off blood for cross matching and place two large-bore IVs. The patient is taken to the operating room. After 4 U of blood are made available in the operating room, you anesthetize him with a rapid sequence technique. He tolerates the anesthetic induction well, and his vital signs remain unchanged. The surgeon cleans the neck and pulls out the wooden knife. There is sudden tachycardia with a dramatic drop in blood pressure. Severe bleeding is seen from the neck wound. The surgeon now does a sternotomy and discovers to everyone's dismay that there is a 0.5–1-cm hole in the aortic arch between the innominate and the left common carotid arteries. Your training dictates that the patient be placed immediately on cardiopulmonary bypass, but you know there is no such thing available. What do you think the surgeon can do to save this patient's life?

Solution

This case happened to a friend of mine. The surgeon clamped the aortic arch proximal to the hole, but in such a way that blood was still flowing through the innominate artery (Fig. 50.1). He started to repair the hole, while at the same time instructing my anesthetic colleague, Dr. Michael Grant, to look for dilatation of the pupils. Michael told him when they started to dilate and then the clamp was let off for a few seconds. This process was completed several times until the hole was repaired. The importance of pupillary dilatation can be argued in this case. I have seen pupils

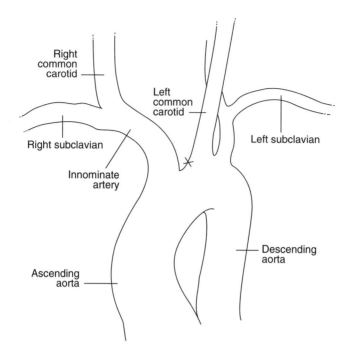

FIGURE 50.1. "X" marks the entry wound of the wooden knife.

dilate dramatically after severe intraoperative bleed, only to return to normal size with adequate resuscitation. Barbiturates could have been used in this case if the patient's blood pressure would have tolerated it.

The patient was taken to the intensive care unit for postoperative ventilation and that is when I met him. Within a few hours, I had removed his endotracheal tube. He made an uneventful recovery.

Discussion

The surgeon was Mr. Rex Henderson FRCS of Empangeni, Natal, South Africa, one of the very best surgeons I have ever had to pleasure to work with. This fellow could do anything. I remember vividly, after he had successfully repaired a severe eye injury, we were called to the scene of an accident where a man was trapped under his tractor. He had lost a lot of blood from a crushed leg and other soft tissue injuries. We were able to place a subclavian IV into the patient while he was upside down. It took some time before we got him to the hospital, but Rex saved the man's leg by repairing the damaged popliteal artery. Later that night we operated on a 1.5-yr-old child that had fallen off a train and needed a hindquarter operation. Rex knew more about pediatric anesthesia than I will never know.

The above patients were saved by a great surgeon and by the presence of a blood bank. But what do you do when you do not have a blood bank? The following story illustrates a remarkable way to solve this problem. During a plenum session in the World Congress of Anesthesiologist in Sidney, Australia, a friend of mine, Brother John from the Australian Franciscan Order, was talking to a large audience about rural anesthesia and trauma. At the time, he was the only doctor working in a large rural area of Borneo. He joked by telling us that he was "the one-armed bandit" (being both the surgeon and the anesthesiologist). When asked what he did when the patients needed blood and he had no blood bank, he said: "That is easy, I am the blood bank. I am O negative." The response of the large audience was total silence – you could hear a pin drop.

Recommendation

Unusual circumstances require unusual methods.

51
An "Old Trick" but a Potential Problem

You have anesthetized an 18-mo-old child with facial deformity requiring surgical correction. He is otherwise healthy and is classified as an American Society of Anesthesiologists physical status 1. Unfortunately, there is more blood loss than anticipated, and the blood pressure is beginning to drop. While awaiting blood from the blood bank, you start infusing albumin 5% (250 ml bottle), but it is going very slowly through your 22-gauge IV in the hand. You have the following options: stop the surgery and get better IV access or aspirate the albumin into a 20-ml syringe from an in-line three-way stopcock, and then turn the stopcock and inject the albumin rapidly into the patient.

Is there another way of getting the albumin quickly into the patient?

Solution

The disposable intravenous administration set for the albumin has an air-vent, which has a one-way valve. By forcing air into the bottle via this valve from a 20-ml syringe, the albumin flows much faster. However, there is a downside to this technique, as air embolism can occur. One must be observant and close the giving set with the IV administration set clamp when the albumin bottle is empty. Not doing this will result in air-embolism. In cases where the albumin administration set has no air vent, a needle with a three-way stopcock and a syringe can produce the same effect.

Discussion

Originally, blood was given from a 500-ml glass bottle. The bottle was hung upside down and a nonvented giving set was inserted through the rubber stop at the neck of the bottle. The blood continued to run out of the bottle because of a small glass tube that went from the neck to nearly the bottom of the bottle. When the blood bottle was turned upside down, there was a connection from the outside to the inside of the bottle above the surface of the blood. In this way, when blood was leaving the bottle, it was replaced with air. Without this small glass tube, blood would not flow out of the bottle. Hence, the "old" way of rapidly infusing blood from the blood bottle was to apply positive pressure, using a sphygmomanometer pump (1). For those of you who have watched the film and TV series M*A*S*H (Mobile Army Service Hospital) from the Korean War, you will have seen this technique being used. I have seen this technique lead to death on an operating table. The anesthesiologist was not paying attention to the fact that the blood had finished being infused and air was rushing in. It was the anesthesiologist's first day on the job. The next day he resigned and left the specialty. Fortunately, blood bottles were replaced in the 1980s with the plastic bags that we now use. Thus, the incidence of air-embolism from this cause has been dramatically reduced.

The disadvantage of the "in-line syringe technique" is that the vein can be damaged by the intermittent pressure exerted on the vein. It can also be messy and time-consuming.

It is important to realize that air embolism can occur from plastic bags, too (2). In this case, air had been noted in a half-filled 6% Hetastarch bag (Abbott Laboratories, North Chicago, IL), but forgotten about when the bag was pressurized. This led to an air embolism in a child with an episode of cardiovascular instability, but no mortality.

Recommendation

Pressurizing, especially an IV bottle, can lead to air embolism. Being vigilant is imperative.

References

1. Bailey H. Pye's Surgical Handicraft. Vol. 1. Bristol: John Wright & Sons Ltd.; 1962:99–101.
2. Balding AM, Roberts JG. Air embolism following infusion of Haemaccel Anaesth Intensive Care 1991;19:130–131.

52
A Loud "Pop" Intraoperatively and Now You Cannot Ventilate

Today, you are to anesthetize a 58-yr-old man, American Society of Anesthesiologists physical status 2, for an anterior resection of a rectal cancer. He is otherwise healthy, but is a big man at 150 kg and 5'8". His airway is classified as a 2. You bring him to the operating room and place him on a "ramp" for easier endotracheal intubation (1). Noninvasive monitors are placed and you anesthetize him in a routine manner. He is easy to ventilate after being given succinylcholine. However, it is a grade 3 view. You place a gum elastic bougie blindly in the trachea and initially try a #9 endotracheal tube (ETT), but it won't go in; neither will a #8 ETT. Eventually, you settle for a #7 ETT. You make a mental note that his trachea must be big because you need to put a much larger than normal air volume into the ETT cuff to prevent a leak. With the airway now secured, the patient is put in a steep Trendelenburg position and the surgery starts. His arms are placed out at 90 degrees from the body and an upper body bear hugger blanket is placed. This is the variety of bear hugger that has sticky sides to the see-through face cover. The operation proceeds uneventfully, until a large "pop" is heard and the bellows of your Narkomed 2B (North American Drager) descend and stay down. You attempt manual ventilation by using the anesthesia machine's collapsible breathing bag. This is unsuccessful. No air fills the bag, even though you use the oxygen flush control button and close off the "pop off valve." You ascertain that the anesthesia hoses are intact and in the correct position. You decide that the loud pop was the bursting of the ETT cuff. You immediately replace the "burst" ETT over a gum elastic bougie with a new one and blow up the cuff. However, there is no improvement. The oxygen saturation is now 76% and the surgeon has stopped working and is looking at you. You have no Ambu bag in the room and you call for one. While waiting, you mouth ventilate through the ETT. It is then that you see the problem. What is it?

Solution

One of the anesthesia breathing hoses coming into the "y" at the patient's mouth looked like it was in place, but in fact it was not. It was barely kept in place with the sticky tape of the bear hugger. Therefore, there was a large leak. When this was fixed the ventilator worked again satisfactorily. The case was completed uneventfully.

Discussion

When this happens, there is only one way to deal with this matter. You disconnect the ETT from the anesthetic tubing at the "y" and do a pressure test. In this way, you can ascertain if it is the circuit or the ETT that is at fault. It is unlikely that both will fail at the same time. If this had been done in the above case, you would have discovered that the leak was in the circuit and not in the ETT. It is so easy to jump to conclusions. Never do that. Always do the pressure test in these cases. It will save you a lot of heart-ache.

Recommendation

There is only one modus operandus when this happens. You must pressurize the anesthetic circuit. In this way you can easily find out if it is the ETT or the circuit that is at fault.

Reference

1. Brodsky JB, Lemmens HJM, Brock-Utne JG, Vierra M, Saidman LJ. Morbid obesity and tracheal intubation. Anesth Analg 2002;94:732–736.

53
Postoperative Median Nerve Injury

You get a call from you orthopedic surgical colleague to say that the patient that you anesthetized for an 11-h spine surgery operation last week has developed a left median nerve conduction block. The diagnosis has been confirmed by a neurologist who is at a loss to find any reason for this. There is no evidence of infection, hematoma, or vascular insufficiency of the hand. The patient has no other problems and is otherwise happy with her surgery. You tell your colleague that you will get back to him. In reviewing your anesthetic record, you see that the anesthetic was uneventful with stable vital signs throughout. Your IV access included two large-bore IVs in the right forearm and the back of right hand. A right subclavian triple-lumen catheter had also been inserted. In addition, she had a left radial intraartery catheter. The arms were both placed forward alongside the head. You go and see the patient and apologize for what has happened. You ask to see her hand. There is nothing abnormal noted with the overlying skin of the left hand and the oxygen saturation reads 100%.

You are at a loss to explain what has occurred. You think the median nerve conduction block should go away and tell the patient so. You have not seen anything like this before.

Can you think of a reason why this has happened to this particular patient?

Solution

It is common practice to hyperextend the wrist during insertion of a radial intraarterial catheter to facilitate arterial puncture and cannulation. Many anesthesiologists leave the wrist in this position for the duration of the surgical procedure, or as long as the catheter is in place. However, it has been shown that wrist hyperextension leads to median nerve conduction block within an average of 43 min (1).

Discussion

Postoperative median nerve injury has, in some cases, been ascribed to direct needle trauma associated with intravenous catheters inserted at the wrist (2). The mechanism of position-related median nerve injury remains undefined, but may be multifactorial (3). In cases where wrist hyperextension is prolonged, it is possible that a stretch-induced focal neuropathy may be the cause (3). In our study (1), we found that wrist hyperextension for arterial line placement and stabilization is likely to result in profound impairment of median nerve function. Although in our study the effects were transient, we believe that prolonged hyperextension may be associated with significant changes in median nerve conduction.

Recommendation

To minimize or prevent median nerve problems in the postoperative period, it is advisable to return the wrist to a neutral position after arterial line placement.

References

1. Chowet AL, Lopes JR, Brock-Utne JG, Jaffe RA. Wrist hyperextension leads to median nerve conduction block. Anesthesiology 2004;100:287–291.
2. Cheney FW, Domino KB, Caplan RA, Posner KL. Nerve injury associated with anesthesia: A closed claim analysis. Anesthesiology 1999;90:1062–1069.
3. Coppieters MW, Van de Velde M, Stappaerts KH. Positioning in anesthesiology: Towards a better understanding of stretch-induced perioperative neuropathies. Anesthesiology 2002;97:75–81.

54
A Patient in a Halo: Watch Out

A 73-yr-old (89 kg and 5'8") female is admitted after a manual vacuum aspiration for surgical stabilization of an unstable cervical neck. You find her in the preoperative holding area, where she is wearing a halo (PMT model 1233, DePuy Spine; The Bremner, Jacksonville, Florida) (Fig. 54.1). The halo is a vest that covers her upper body and shoulders. The halo is attached to the head on both sides of the skull with adjustable headlocks. These can be adjusted in three ways: A/P positioning, flexion/extension, and traction/distraction. You manage to examine her chest with your stethoscope, although this is not easy due to the vest that is covering her back and the front of the chest. You are comforted that the chest x-ray taken 1 h ago is normal. She has no other health problems. She tells you that she underwent an elective cholecystectomy 6 mo previously under general anesthesia without any problems. She can open her mouth and you can clearly see her uvula. She is very nervous and does not want a fiberoptic endotracheal intubation. You say you will put her to sleep and secure the airway after she is asleep. She is very grateful. You induce anesthesia in a routine manner and find that you can easily place a #7 endotracheal tube (ETT) in the trachea with a MacIntosh #3 blade. You have a grade 1 view. The operation concludes satisfactorily within 2 h, and the patient wakes up still in the halo. As she follows commands and is breathing adequately, you remove the ETT from the trachea. You take her to the recovery room, where, initially, her vital signs are within normal limits. You are next door in the preoperative holding area talking to the next patient, when a nurse tells you to come quickly to the recovery room as your halo case is not breathing and her oxygen saturation is 87%. You run to see the patient. A nurse is attempting to mask ventilate the patient with no success, despite using a Guedel's airway. You ask for and get a MacIntosh #3 blade and insert the blade into the mouth of the now semiunconscious woman, but to your dismay you see nothing. You ascertain that this is indeed a MacIntosh #3 blade and try again, but again you see nothing. You secure the airway by blindly passing a bougie into the trachea. You are at a loss to understand why, within 2.5 h, with no evidence of airway edema, you now can see nothing during

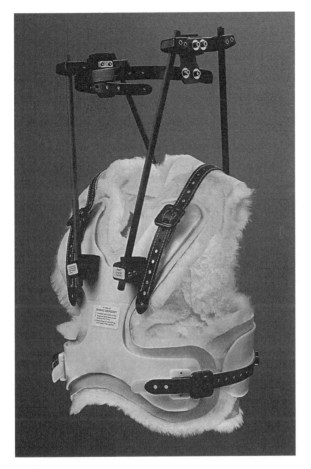

FIGURE 54.1. A picture of the PMT model 1233, DePuy Spine. With permission from The Bremer, Jacksonville, FL.

laryngoscopy, whereas previously you had a grade 1 view. What do you think the problem is?

Solution

Unbeknownst to you, the surgeon adjusted the headblocks forward so that the anatomy of the airway changed. Now you have no view of the vocal cords.

Discussion

When a patient is wearing a halo, it is important to ascertain if the halo has been changed during surgery. If it has been, you cannot presume that you will be able to reintubate the trachea easily. Being aware of this problem is imperative for the patient's safety. It may be prudent to leave a bougie in place when you remove the ETT from the trachea, especially if there is a possibility that the surgeon may have moved the halo during the surgery.

Recommendation

Be aware that a surgeon may not tell you that he has adjusted the halo position. The result of this adjustment may be that a patient with a grade 1 airway during induction of anesthesia has a very different, and potentially difficult, airway after surgery.

55
Now or Never: Developing Professional Judgment

You have started a new job as an anesthesiologist in private practice. Your first case on your first day seems a simple one. The patient is a 27-yr-old male (weight 90 kg and height 5′8″) scheduled for elective arthroscopy of shoulder, knee, and ankle, all on the left side. He is an unmarried construction worker accompanied by his father. He is a motorbike fanatic and has fallen off his bike in the past. He claims he is perfectly healthy except that in the last 6 mo he has developed a hoarseness of his voice. He tells you that it has not gotten worse. His father nods in agreement. He went to an ear, nose, and throat (ENT) surgeon 3 mo ago, who told him that he has vocal cord polyps. The ENT surgeon indicated that there was no problem. However, you do not agree and you speak to the orthopedic surgeon to relay your concern. You suggest that a new ENT consult be obtained and that his operation be canceled today. The surgeon informs you that it is "now or never" for this surgery, as the patient's insurance expires tomorrow. You consider regional blocks, but the patient refuses them and states he wants to be asleep. He would rather leave without the surgery than having it done under regional blocks. If you decided to go ahead with a general anesthetic, how would you do it for this patient, remembering that he has to be on right-side down for the shoulder surgery?

Solution

The best solution is to cancel the case. However, this happened to me on my first day in private practice and this is what I did. Because the patient wanted the surgery, I warned him and his father that going ahead with a general anesthetic could result in a tracheotomy, and/or postoperative ventilation in an intensive care unit for maybe a day or two, or even death. I wrote that in the chart and had them sign my note. In a court of law I don't think it makes much difference, but it made me feel better. In the preoperative holding area I gave him atropine 0.5 mg IV to reduce salivary secretions, together with midazolam 6 mg IV. He was taken to the operating room (OR) and noninvasive monitors were placed. After a smooth IV induction with propofol, a #3 laryngeal mask airway (LMA) was inserted. He was positioned on the OR table with his right side down. Ventilation was manually assisted throughout the shoulder surgery. When the surgery was completed, the patient was placed on his back and spontaneous ventilation resumed. At the completion of the surgery, the LMA was removed while the patient was still asleep. He made an uneventful recovery and was discharged home the same day.

Discussion

This is a difficult case to manage. The correct thing to do is to cancel; however, when "forced" to do the case, regional blocks would have been a good option. But again, an overdose of local anesthetic, with respiratory/cardiac arrest, could have proven disastrous. I elected not to place an endotracheal tube (ETT) because that could have made the polyps bleed or have caused other problems. Using a fiberoptic scope to look at the vocal cords before anesthesia would not be of any use either, as in a court of law the question would be "How many vocal cord polyps have you seen," and so on.

Recommendation

Always do what is best for the patient and don't take risks. In this case, a risk was taken, but I was fortunate that the outcome was a good one for the patient.

56
General Anesthesia in a Patient with Chronic Amphetamine Use

You are assigned to anesthetize a 59-yr-old female for a total hip replacement. Her history is significant for depression and she has taken dextroamphetamine 15 mg b.d. for over 3 yr. Would you proceed or would you recommend discontinuing amphetamine therapy before general anesthesia, and thereby delay the surgery?

Solution

We have recently reported nine cases of patients taking chronic prescription of amphetamines who underwent general anesthesia and had a safe outcome (1,2). The conclusions suggest potential stable anesthesia management in patients on chronic prescription amphetamines. However, it is recommended that direct-acting vasopressors, including phenylephrine or epinephrine, should be readily available intraoperatively. In the nine cases above, none required any vasopressor drugs.

Discussion

Amphetamines are noncatecholamines, which are sympathetic amines with powerful central nervous system stimulation activity. Their action is thought to be associated with the local release of biogenic amines, such as norepinephrine, from nerve-terminal storage sites (3). Peripheral actions from amphetamine include an increase of systolic and diastolic blood pressure and a weak bronchodilator and respiratory stimulant action. Chronic amphetamine exposure with stimulation of the adrenergic and peripheral nerve terminals causes a depletion of catecholamine receptor storage (4). This reduction in catecholamine, especially norepinephrine, is thought to contribute to a blunted physiologic and sympathetic response to hypotension, as has been reported in anesthesia (5,6). Hence, intraoperative refractory hypotension with or without bradycardia in patients taking amphetamines should be treated with direct-acting vasopressors, such as epinephrine (50–100 mg IV) or phenylephrine (50–100 mg IV). Ephedrine has been reported to have a decreased or absent pressor response after chronic amphetamine use (6). The single case report, in 1979 (5), of cardiac arrest and death during a cesarean delivery in a chronic amphetamine abuser has become the reference in the anesthetic literature to warn against the use of general anesthesia in these cases. It is interesting to note that the authors (5) admit that it was difficult to prove the association of the patient's drug use and the general anesthesia, as there were other concurrent clinical factors that could have contributed to her demise. Unfortunately, the case report has been incorporated in many anesthesia textbooks, and has thereby contributed to the belief that amphetamines must and should be discontinued prior to general anesthesia and surgery to avoid patient morbidity and mortality.

In our two reports (1,2) dealing with nine elective surgical patients in which the amphetamine was not stopped preoperatively, the general anesthesia proceeded successfully with no cardiovascular instability in any of the patients. No dramatic fluctuations in arterial blood pressures were observed at induction or during the course of the surgeries that necessitated the use of pressor treatment.

Recommendation

We believe that patients on chronic amphetamines may not need to discontinue the drug before elective surgery, but that direct-acting vasopressors should be readily available intraoperatively.

References

1. Healzer JM, Fisher SP, Brook MW, Brock-Utne JG. General anesthesia is a patient on long-term amphetamine therapy: Is there cause for concern? Anesth Analg 2000;91:758–759.
2. Fisher SP, Schmiesing CA, Guta CG, Brock-Utne JG. General anesthesia and chronic amphetamine use. Should the drug be stopped preoperatively? Anesth Analg 2006;103:203–206.
3. Carr LA, Moore KE. Norepinephrine release from brain by d-amphetamine in vivo. Science 1969;164:322–323.
4. Hardman JG, Limbird LE. Amphetamine: The pharmacological basis of therapeutics. 1996;219–221.
5. Samuels SI, Maze A. Albright G. Cardiac arrest during cesarean section a chronic amphetamine abuser. Anesth Analg 1979;58:528–530.
6. Johnston RR, Way WL, Miller RD. Alteration of anesthetic requirements by amphetamine. Anesthesiology 1972;36:357–363.

57
What Is Wrong with This Picture?

You are sent to investigate an increased incidence of difficult endotracheal intubations in a mission hospital in Africa. On the first morning you are there, you observe an anesthesiologist giving a general anesthetic to a patient for an elective cesarean section. A rapid sequence induction with etomidate and succinylcholine is followed by the insertion of a MacIntosh blade #3 inserted into the mouth and larynx using the left hand. What follows then is contra to everything you have ever seen before. The anesthesiologist, instead of placing the endotracheal tube (ETT) to the right of the blade and into the trachea, places his right hand over the left hand and guides the ETT successfully into the trachea. You are amazed, but after careful inspection of the blade you understand the reason for this unorthodox way of placing the ETT in the trachea.

Without seeing the blade what will you say the problem could be?

Solution

A left-handed laryngoscope blade for left handed anesthesiologists (Figs. 57.1 and 57.2).

Discussion

This happened to a friend of mine, Dr. Mannie Mankowitz, in the 1970s. He never tired of telling the story. The interesting part of the story was that this was the only blade they had in the hospital. It had been donated by a left-handed anesthesiologist who no longer worked there. Please remember that a very high percentage of anesthetics in many parts of Africa is provided

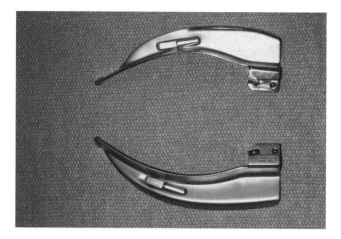

FIGURE 57.1. The left handed laryngoscopy blade is on the bottom.

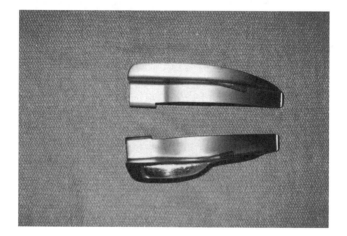

FIGURE 57.2. The left handed laryngoscopy blade is on the bottom.

by health care workers who are neither doctors nor nurses, and with a minimal amount of training.

Recommendation

Be aware that there are left-handed laryngoscopes.

58
The One-Eyed Patient

A 78-yr-old female is scheduled for a right upper lobectomy under general anesthesia. She is 54 kg and 5′10″ tall. Her weight has been steady for as long as she can remember. Her history is significant for hypertension, a 50-yr smoking history, and an enucleation of the right eye for tumor 10 yr ago. She is unsure what the tumor was. She has a glass eye, but prefers to wear a large black eye patch that covers the whole orbit, including the eyebrow. Otherwise, her medical history and physical exam are unremarkable. She has a class 2 airway. After sedation with midazolam 1 mg IV, she is taken to the operating room where a routine general anesthetic, with fentanyl, thiopental, and vecuronium, is induced uneventfully. Mask ventilation with sevoflurane in 100% oxygen proves to be difficult, as there is a large leak detected around her face. A larger and well-inflated facemask is placed over her mouth and nose, but a large leak is still present. By increasing the fresh gas flow to 12 liters, the patient is easy to ventilate, but the leak is still present and everyone in the room can smell the sevoflurane. You again perform a pressure leak test on the anesthetic absorber circuit (you did it before you started), but you find nothing wrong. Another anesthesiologist is brought in to hold the mask with both hands while you elect to ventilate the patient with the reservoir bag. Despite this the leak is still there. Her vital signs remain stable, but you are concerned, as this unexplained leak is something you have not encountered before. What will you do now?

Solution

Remove the eye patch and, in this case, you see the orbital cavity without a glass eye. The reason for the leak is now quiet apparent as there is an anatomical passage from the mouth cavity to the orbit of the eye. Having discovered the cause of the leak, tracheal intubation with a double-lumen tube is done atraumatically on the first attempt with the patient fully paralyzed. The operation proceeds uneventfully and she is discharged home after 4 d in hospital.

Discussion

This is the only case like this I have seen (1). At the time, we were at complete loss as to the cause of the large leak. If the patient had been bigger, with or without lung pathology, mask oxygenation of the patient could have been a real problem. A 4-in vaginal pack, made moist with water, could have been packed into the orbit to minimize the leak.

Recommendation

Be aware of the patient with an eye patch. Should it be difficult to mask ventilate due to a large orbital leak, a moist vaginal pack can be used.

Reference

1. Brock-Utne JG. Beware of the patient with an eye patch. Anesth Analg. 2007;104:1615.

59
A Near Tragedy

After a long week in the operating room, you are relaxing on a beach south of Durban in South Africa. The weather is wonderful. Just behind the beach is a lagoon. When the tide is coming in, the Indian Ocean enters the lagoon at the end of the beach where there are many rocks. Suddenly, there is a cry for help, and you rush to the rocks to see a 6-yr-old boy in the water to his armpits with the tide coming in. He is screaming that he cannot get his foot out. Two men are both busy trying to release his foot. It will not come out. Over 200 people are now gathered around. You introduce yourself, offer help, as an anesthesiologist, to the two men, and discover that one is an orthopedic surgeon and the other a cardiac surgeon. They say they may need your help, as in less than 10–15 minutes the water will be over the boy's head and in that case, they will need to amputate the foot. You run to your car. In the boot, you have all the anesthetic drugs and equipment (including a draw-over vaporizer) you will need to anesthetize the child. You consider sedating the child with the drugs you have in your bag, namely meperidine, fentanyl, or morphine but are concerned they may not suffice in preventing pain and you may also loose the airway. The other option is a general anesthesia with propofol, succinylcholine, an endotracheal tube, and a draw-over vaporizer. Is there any other drug or technique you would consider?

Solution

This happened to me. The beach was South Broom at Easter and the year was 1980. An unknown orthopedic surgeon and the thoracic surgeon Dr. Bruce Henderson (no relation of Rex Henderson of Empangeni, who is mentioned in Chapter 50) and I were left with this dilemma. The child was given ketamine 6 mg/kg intramuscularly. This gave him sufficient pain relief for the surgeons to remove the foot intact while I looked after his airway. With the patient breathing spontaneously and with no sign of pain, the foot came out, but badly bruised and bleeding. Happily, the child made an uneventful recovery.

Recommendation

When living in remote places, always carry adequate medical equipment with you if you feel that you would like to render medical help. If you want to assist, you will never know when you will need it. Shortly after arriving in South Africa, I was called to help a neighbor who had collapsed. I came with my normal GP bag, which had no laryngoscope or endotracheal tubes, facemasks, or Ambu bag. I found myself hopelessly unprepared. If I had been able to control his airway properly, I might have saved his life. As it was, the patient died. It was very distressing. Shortly after that, I invested in a Laerdal bag with laryngoscopes, endotracheal tubes, IVs, etc. I always carried it in the trunk of my car and have used it at least 9–10 times over a period of 17 yr. The chest drain, which I had, was used only once. You do not want to be caught out like a carpenter without his tools.

Lastly, always think outside the box. Ketamine, in this case, was a foot-saver.

60
Robot-Assisted Surgery:
A Word of Caution

Today, you are anesthetizing a 3-mo-old, 6.1 kg infant with biliary atresia. The operation is scheduled for laparoscopic Kasai using a robot-assisted surgical system. The system consists of a remote operating console and a wide-base surgical cart. Inhaled anesthesia with sevoflurane, peripheral IV access, securing the airway with an endotracheal tube, and a radial line inserted in the operating room (OR). The endotracheal tube position is confirmed by auscultation, and a precordial stethoscope is placed over the patient's left chest. An orogastric tube is used to decompress the stomach. The patient is elevated approximately 4 in off the OR table on blankets and an egg crate to allow the greatest range of motion for the robotic arms. The OR table is positioned in a 30 degree reverse Trendelenburg to facilitate surgical exposure. The operation proceeds with placement of the robotic cart and arms. Thirty minutes into the case, there is a gradual drop in blood pressure. There is no obvious bleeding, but you are concerned. A medical student suggests that you put the patient in Trendelenburg, as he observes that the child has his feet down. Is this a good idea?

Solution

No, this is not a good idea. If you are to change the OR table in these cases, the robotic instruments must be disengaged (1). The reason is that the robotic arms are solid structures, and moving the patient with the robot and its appendages in place can and will cause major injuries to the patient. In case of an airway emergency or severe hypotension or cardiac arrest, resuscitation of the patient requires that the robotic instruments are quickly removed.

Discussion

For the patient to be safe during robot-assisted surgery, advanced planning is essential as to what to do should a problem arise. All team members must familiarize themselves with the issues that are specific for this type of surgery. The biggest problem with these robots is that access to the patient is severely limited. It is essential that the OR team practice the crisis scenario of removing the robotic equipment and gaining access to the patient quickly, should it be necessary. The limited access to the patient requires special monitoring. A left-sided precordial stethoscope can monitor inadvertent right mainstem intubation. Core temperature should be monitored and maintained with a warm OR, warm IV fluid, and forced air warming. The latter can be difficult to place because of the need for surgical access and the placement of the robotic arm. The placement of an intraarterial catheter allows for continuous arterial blood pressure monitoring and blood gas sampling. The latter is important, as the laparoscopic operations lead to decrease in lung volumes, impaired ventilation, and increased CO_2 absorption (1).

In this case, an inadvertent gradual increase in pneumoperitoneum decreased venous return. When this was corrected, the child's blood pressure returned to normal. It is also important to realize that with the use of the reverse Trendelenburg position, a 50% reduction in cardiac index can be expected (2).

Recommendation

Advanced planning and understanding of the robot equipment is essential before anesthetizing a patient undergoing robot-assisted surgery. Failure to do so can lead to disaster.

References

1. Mariano ER, Furukawa L, Woo RK, Albanese CT, Brock-Utne JG. Anesthesia concerns for robot-assisted laparoscopy in an infant. Anesth Analg 2004;99:1665–1667.
2. Joris JL, Noirot DP, Legrand MJ, et al. Hemodynamic changes during laparoscopic cholecystectomy. Anesth Analg 1993;76:1067–1071.

61
An Airway Emergency in an Out of Hospital Surgical Office

Today you find yourself in a freestanding oral surgery office that is 3 miles from the nearest hospital. You are to provide conscious sedation for a 38-yr-old man, (80 kg and 5′10″). He is scheduled for a 3-hr oral surgery procedure, consisting of multiple dental extractions, alveoloplasty, and placement of multiple dental implants in the mandible. He is otherwise healthy and classified as an American Society of Anesthesiologists physical status 1. The conscious sedation consists of midazolam, ketamine, meperidine, and propofol in multiple divided doses. He is monitored using standard monitoring, including a precordial stethoscope. Supplemental oxygen is provided throughout the procedure via a nasal cannula. After 2.5 h of an uneventful surgical procedure, the surgeon notices a rapidly expanding hematoma in the floor of the mouth, as well as a rapid enlargement of the posterior part of the tongue. The patient begins to complain of difficulty in breathing. His oxygen saturation remains in the mid 90s. The surgeon's attempt to control the bleeding fails. He now believes the reason for the hematomas is an arterial bleed in the floor of the mouth caused by one of the implants. The hematoma continues to expand, and the saturation is now falling to 85%. You stop all IV sedation, attempt a blind nasal intubation, and provide a jaw thrust with a facemask, but no improvement is seen. Any attempt at an laryngeal mask airway insertion or oral intubation is deemed impossible due to the degree of mechanical obstruction caused by the hematoma. What is the most important thing to do now, and what other airway maneuvers can you think of?

Solution

The first thing to do is to call 911 so that you can get the patient transported to a hospital. As for the airway, sit the patient up and place bilateral French nasal airways. But most importantly, place a tongue suture to retract the tongue. This should help alleviate the airway obstruction.

However tongue suture may be difficult to place after the hematoma has already developed. Hence the placement of a tongue suture prophylactically, in cases where a lot of surgery is anticipated, is advisable.

Discussion

This problem happened to a friend of mine, Dr. Terri Homer. In her case, the surgeon had placed the tongue suture at an earlier stage of the procedure. The paramedics arrived within 5 min and the patient was transported to the hospital via an ambulance in a sitting position, with nasal airways and with Dr. Homer maintaining constant forward retraction of the tongue with the tongue suture. This airway management maintained the oxygen saturation in the low 90s. On arrival in the hospital emergency room, the ear, nose, and throat team was called. A successful fiberoptic nasal intubation was performed. The patient was sedated and taken to the operating room, where he underwent surgery with successful control of the arterial bleeding of the floor of the mouth. Postoperatively, the patient remained intubated overnight in the intensive care unit and was discharged from the hospital 48 h later.

If the airway had been lost despite the maneuvers mentioned above, then a cricothyrotomy kit should be available. Failing that, then a tracheostomy must be done. It is also important to know that many dental surgeons place a tongue suture (under local anesthesia) at the beginning of the procedure, which is used to intermittently/continuously gently retract the tongue during the surgery. As the IV sedation is given intermittently, there may be occasional respiratory obstruction that can easily be treated with a gentle pressure on the tongue suture.

Recommendation

Remember and know the various options that you have available to you to manage a rapidly obstructing airway in the out of hospital surgical setting. Also remember to call 911, as soon as you realize you have an airway problem.

62
Bonus Question: Is the Patient Paralyzed?

You have anesthetized, in a routine manner, a 30-yr-old man American Society of Anesthesiologists physical status 2 who is scheduled for a cervical lymph node biopsy with a possible neck dissection. Succinylcholine 70 mg is given because the surgeon has requested no muscle relaxation during surgery. Ten minutes later the surgeon, with his finger in the patient's mouth, asks you if the patient is paralyzed. How can you best convince him that the patient is not paralyzed?

Solution/Discussion

Dr. Michael Keating and I were faced with this question by a surgeon (1). It was quickly answered as Michael activated the nerve stimulator, which was placed over the trigeminal nerve. Immediately, the patient closed his mouth firmly. Thus, the surgeon was assured that the patient was no longer paralyzed, but he did complain of a sore finger.

Recommendation

We published this finding (1) and asked the question: "Have we found another use for the nerve stimulator?"

Reference

1. Keating M, Brock-Utne JG. Another use for the nerve stimulator? Anesth Analg 1995;81:1312.

Appendix
Technique for Making a Quick Underwater Drain

1. Cut a primary IV set in half.
2. Insert the piercing pin of the primary IV set into a 250/500 ml container of IV fluid after having removed the white stopper.
3. The cut end of the primary IV set (with the Cair clamp) is inserted into the fluid through the outlet of the plastic container that you have pierced (See Step 1). The end of the primary IV set tubing is introduced well below the fluid level.
4. The proximal end of the 14-G catheter, after it is inserted into the pleural cavity, is then attached to the male adaptor on the primary IV set.
5. An 18-G needle is inserted through the drip injection port of the plastic container to act as a vent.

Index

Printed in the United States of America